DEATH AND MEDICAL POWER
An Ethical Analysis of Dutch Euthanasia Practice

HENK A. M. J. TEN HAVE
and
JOS V. M. WELIE

Open University Press
McGraw-Hill Education
McGraw-Hill House
Shoppenhangers Road
Maidenhead
Berkshire
England
SL6 2QL

email: enquiries@openup.co.uk
world wide web: www.openup.co.uk

and Two Penn Plaza, New York, NY 10121–2289, USA

First published 2005

A catalogue record of this book is available from the British Library

ISBN-10: 0 335 21755 9 (pb) 0 335 21756 7(hb)
ISBN-13: 978 0335 217557 (pb) 978 0335 21756 4(hb)

Library of Congress Cataloging-in-Publication Data
CIP data applied for

Cover image: Reconstruction drawing (fragment) of the late medieval 'Dance with Death' fresco in the St Marien Church (Berlin, Germany).

Typeset by YHT Ltd, London
Printed in Poland by OZGraf S.A. www.polskabook.pl

DEATH A D CLINICAL
POWER

FACING DEATH

Series editor: David Clark, Professor of Medical Sociology,
University of Lancaster

The subject of death in late modern culture has become a rich field of theoretical, clinical and policy interest. Widely regarded as a taboo until recent times, death now engages a growing interest among social scientists, practitioners and those responsible for the organization and delivery of human services. Indeed, how we die has become a powerful commentary on how we live and the specialized care of dying people holds an important place within modern health and social care.

This series captures such developments. Among the contributors are leading experts in death studies, from sociology, anthropology, social psychology, ethics, nursing, medicine and pastoral care. A particular feature of the series is its attention to the developing field of palliative care, viewed from the perspectives of practitioners, planners and policy analysts; here several authors adopt a multidisciplinary approach, drawing on recent research, policy and organizational commentary, and reviews of evidence-based practice. Written in a clear, accessible style, the entire series will be essential reading for students of death, dying and bereavement, and for anyone with an involvement in palliative care research, service delivery or policymaking.

Current and forthcoming titles:

David Clark, Jo Hockley and Sam Ahmedzai (eds): *New Themes in Palliative Care*
David Clark and Jane E. Seymour: *Reflections on Palliative Care*
David Clark and Michael Wright: *Transitions in End of Life Care: Hospice and Related Developments in Eastern Europe and Central Asia*
Mark Cobb: *The Dying Soul: Spiritual Care at the End of Life*
Kirsten Costain Schou and Jenny Hewison: *Experiencing Cancer: Quality of Life in Treatment*
David Field, David Clark, Jessica Corner and Carol Davis (eds): *Researching Palliative Care*
Anne Grinyer: *Cancer in Young Adults: Through Parents' Eyes*
Henk ten Have and David Clark (eds): *The Ethics of Palliative Care: European Perspectives*
Henk ten Have and Jos Welie: *Death and Medical Power: An Ethical Analysis of Dutch Euthanasia Practice*
Jenny Hockey, Jeanne Katz and Neil Small (eds): *Grief, Mourning and Death Ritual*
Jo Hockley and David Clark (eds): *Palliative Care for Older People in Care Homes*
David W. Kissane and Sidney Bloch: *Family Focused Grief Therapy*
Gordon Riches and Pam Dawson: *An Intimate Loneliness: Supporting Bereaved Parents and Siblings*
Lars Sandman: *A Good Death: On the Value of Death and Dying*
Jane E. Seymour: *Critical Moments: Death and Dying in Intensive Care*
Anne-Mei The: *Palliative Care and Communication: Experiences in the Clinic*
Tony Walter: *On Bereavement: The Culture of Grief*
Simon Woods: *Death's Dominion: Ethics at the End of Life*

Contents

Series editor's preface

The Facing Death series has a strong commitment to exploring some of the more challenging issues that surround end of life care in our society. Of these, none is more controversial, complex or frequently misunderstood as that form of legalised, medical killing that we have come to call euthanasia. In recent times the country that has attracted most attention in these debates is of course the Netherlands, where euthanasia has been more openly practiced, first as a decriminalised activity and then as an action legal in the sight of the law, if subject to particular guidelines and procedures.

This new addition to the series is therefore most welcome. Henk ten Have and Jos Welie have spent two decades observing and studying the Dutch euthanasia scene. They bring to their subject matter the analytic powers of bioethics and moral philosophy, coupled with skilled historical and socio-cultural observation. They take us through a comprehensive account of cases, debates and practices surrounding euthanasia in the Netherlands, beginning with the famous Postma case of 1971 and moving through to the enactment of new legislation in 2002. Their thesis is challenging. Seeing euthanasia as initially a reaction to medical dominance at the end of life, they argue that, paradoxically, its legalisation in the Netherlands has led to an unprecedented increase in medical power over life, unparalleled in the history of medicine and indeed exceeding that of the modern state itself. They point to the profusion of definitions, criteria and justifications for euthanasia that have been shifting and altering on a frequent basis over the last three decades. They suggest that this is itself evidence of an inadequate theoretical basis for the justification of euthanasia, making it subject to a raft of changing empirical and contingent influences. Their detailed description of these processes makes compelling reading.

Death and Medical Power adds to several other volumes in the Facing Death series that focus on ethical and moral issues in care at the end of life. It can be read alongside Ten Have and Clark's collection on the ethics of palliative care in Europe[1] as well as Sandman's volume on the good death[2]. It also relates to some of the debates explored by Clark and Seymour in their sociological and policy analysis of palliative care[3]. This book on the Dutch experience of euthanasia deserves to be widely read by all of those engaged in thinking and practice surrounding contemporary end of life care. It challenges a number of entrenched assumptions and will doubtless provoke further discussion and debate. It is a worthy addition to the Facing Death series and deserves to be widely read.

David Clark
February 2005

1. Have, H. ten and Clark, D. (2002) The *Ethics of Palliative Care: European Perspectives*. Buckingham: Open University Press.
2. Sandman, L. (2005) A *Good Death* Maidenhead: Open University Press.
3. Clark, D. and Seymour, J. (1999) *Reflections on Palliative Care*. Buckingham: Open University Press.

Introduction

To many people, the Netherlands is identified with tulips, windmills and legalized mercy killing. Advocates as well as opponents view the Dutch practice as an important experiment, the results of which will prove the important benefits or inevitable dangers of euthanasia and physician assisted suicide.

From an argumentative perspective, it would appear that advocates of euthanasia can make a stronger case. First, euthanasia is between the physician and patient only. Unlike abortion, there is no third person involved who is unable to defend himself yet whose life is at stake. Second, euthanasia and assisted suicide is about patient choice. There now is widespread agreement that patients have the right to determine which medical treatments to undergo and which to refuse, even if such refusal implies death. Third, physicians are best able to counsel terminally ill patients about their prognosis and remaining therapeutical options, such that the patient's choice to leave life is really an informed choice. Finally, it is only fair that the medical system, which created these situations of unbearable suffering by keeping patients alive with drugs and technologies, also offer patients a way out, a humane and dignified exit. Thus all important principles of medical ethics are fulfilled. First, nobody is being harmed. Second, patient autonomy is respected. Third, the patient's best interests are fostered. Finally, legalization of euthanasia restores justice.

Unable to deny the apparent validity of these arguments in favour of legalized euthanasia and physician assisted suicide, opponents of euthanasia frequently resort to scare tactics. Once assisted suicide and voluntary euthanasia are accepted and have become common, society will move towards mercy killing of demented patients; the mentally handicapped will be next; then disabled newborns; and soon every terminally ill patient will be a potential candidate for euthanasia. But even if historical and socio-logical evidence could be mounted to make such a slippery slope likely, it is at best a prudential argument. It would imply that we should be very cautious when legalizing physician assisted suicide and euthanasia. But it does not invalidate the ethical arguments themselves in favour of eutha-nasia as summarized above. The same is true of the alleged danger that patients could become victims of impatient physicians or family members who callously believe the patient's death is overdue. Even if opponents could present evidence of the existence of such evil caregivers, surely such exceptions do not invalidate the ideals sketched above. Granted, the med-ical profession must seriously guard against physicians' misusing their power and the public's trust vested in them. But that is true of all medical practice, and that is why medicine is a profession, a self-disciplining occupation.

If only euthanasia were a clear indicator of society's courting Nazism; if only euthanasia were the prerogative of mal-intended physicians, it would be easy to oppose mercy killing. But the Dutch experiment does not support such charges. Indeed, among our best colleagues and dearest friends are physicians who have practised euthanasia. The apparent strength of the case in favour of euthanasia and the apparent weakness of the arguments against have resulted in ever more judicial lenience towards Dutch physi-cians who violated the legal prohibition against euthanasia and assisted suicide. It finally led to the legalization of these practices. Belgium has since followed suit; the US state of Oregon legalized physician assisted suicide; and several other US states have come close to doing so. Elsewhere in the world, the possibility of decriminalization is likewise being entertained and studied.

What seems to have escaped most participants in and observers of the Dutch experiment is its paradoxical nature. And paradoxes should always invoke concern, among opponents and advocates alike. What paradox are we referring to? As we will explain in great detail in this book, the push towards legalized euthanasia has been spurred on by the rapid growth of medical power, or rather the dissatisfaction with that growth. Physicians had always been prominent figures in society, playing a dominant and at times decisive role in people's lives. But this power was largely fictitious, based on pretentious claims of healing abilities, not on actual abilities. In the course of the twentieth century, this situation changed dramatically. Scientific and technological advances provided physicians with the actual ability to protect life effectively and extend it significantly. Medical power had become real. Indeed, to many it had become all too real. The newly gained power of physicians to keep patients alive seemingly for ever resulted in a call to empower patients instead. Legalized euthanasia and assisted suicide were – and continue to be – seen as prime examples of patient empowerment.

But immediately a paradox began to take hold. Instead of curbing medical power, these developments expanded it. From the very beginning, physicians managed to claim a monopoly on euthanasia and assistance in suicide. The Dutch courts followed suit and granted legal immunity only to physicians. Dutch parliament likewise agreed and has allowed only physicians to assist in patients' suicide or commit euthanasia. Elsewhere in the world, physicians have also been granted a monopoly as most aptly reflected in the standard English acronym PAS, physician assisted suicide. Thus, after three decades of combating the ever-increasing medicalization of society and the power of the medical profession to orchestrate people's lives, medical power has only augmented with the power to procure death. Nobody in Dutch society has such awesome, legally sanctioned power: only physicians.

In subsequent chapters we will show that this power is very real indeed. For all the talk about patient autonomy, the actual decision makers are physicians. And this should worry all of us, opponents and advocates of euthanasia alike. It should worry us because this increase in power has not been the result of a coup by a small minority of megalomaniac physicians. Nor are the rising costs of health care causing an economically depressed Dutch society to flirt with fascist solutions. If only things were that simple. We will show that the paradox evoked by the practice of a 'good death' can be explained only by its underlying philosophy of a good life. More specifically, the decisive justification of euthanasia practice is not patient self-determination. It is the quality of patients' lives, or rather the alleged lack thereof.

Our examination of the practice of mercy killing in the Netherlands has rendered us forceful opponents thereof. This book hence is not a value-neutral description of the Dutch experiment. Although we have tried to do justice to the arguments in favour, we readily admit that this book argues against medical engagement in and legalization of mercy killing. Nevertheless, we hope that advocates of euthanasia will read it. For we do agree with their premise that medicine's newly gained power to extend life is a mixed blessing. We have to find a way to provide patients not with a 'good death' but with a 'good dying process'. We therefore interweave in our critical examination of Dutch euthanasia practice an ardent plea in favour of palliative care. We will show that such an approach ethically is both different from and preferable to medically procured death. Thus it is fitting that our book is part of a series on palliative care and we thank the series editor for including it.

This book is the result of two decades of studying the ethical and legal aspects of euthanasia and physician assisted suicide. We have only gained a better insight into the complexities of this practice because so many colleagues have helped us understand the many ethical subtleties and distinctions. Two decades of such discussions means too many names to list.

We can only hope that this book will help others gain some clarity as well, and particularly those among our readers who actually provide care to terminally ill patients. For in the end it is up to them to make sure that our time of dying, a time that will come for all of us, will be good.

Finally, we would like to thank our academic institutions for stimulating us to examine such important bioethical issues regarding the end of life: the Department of Ethics, Philosophy and History of Medicine (University Medical Center Nijmegen, the Netherlands), and the Center for Health Policy and Ethics (Creighton University Medical Center, USA). The views expressed in this book do not in any way reflect the views of these universities or of UNESCO with which one of the authors is presently affiliated.

Euthanasia and medical power

The Postma case

There was no alternative. Five months earlier she had suffered a stroke. Although the treatment in the Assen hospital had resulted in a gradual improvement of her condition, she continued to suffer from partial paralysis and problems with her speech. Mrs van Boven-Grevelink could not return home. She needed permanent care. So she was transferred to a Catholic nursing clinic in Oosterwolde, a small village in the northern Dutch province of Friesland.

Unfortunately the transfer turned out to have a detrimental effect on her condition. One of her two daughters, visiting her on the first day, was shocked to see her mother in a confused and absent-minded state, unable to communicate. Mrs van Boven's condition continued to fluctuate during the ensuing days. She remained wheelchair-bound, had difficulties in hearing and talking, and could not move her left arm. She had lost interest in the people around her, her family and grandchildren. Often she recognized her daughters, mentioned their names, and repeated that she wanted them to leave. At times, she even told them that she no longer wanted to see them.

One day in October, her daughters found her tied up in bed with the bed rails raised. She was pale and her face covered with bandages. It turned out that she had fallen out of bed. A few days later, she explained that she had thrown herself out of the bed deliberately in a primitive attempt to kill herself. She repeatedly told her daughters that she did not want to be in this situation, that she wanted 'something to die'.

Approximately one month after her transfer to Oosterwolde, the nursing clinic physician was informed by the head nurse that Mrs van Boven was dying. This deterioration in her condition was unusually sudden, for only an hour earlier a laboratory analyst had visited Mrs van Boven to take a blood sample for a haemoglobin test; he had entertained a normal conversation with the patient. However, so the nurse explained, there was no need to hurry; Mrs van Boven was in the company of one of her daughters and son-in-law.

In fact, this daughter was a physician, and so was her husband, Dr Postma. Both had been working as family practitioners in Noordwolde, a village not far from Oosterwolde. The Postmas had come to the conclusion that Mother was lacking the will to live ever since she had been hospitalized in Assen. Several times Mother had blamed the medical doctors, and her own medical family members in particular, for having saved her life. She had always been fond of life, but also stubborn and unwilling to make compromises. Being conscious and competent, she had realized that she was disabled and unlikely to recover. Nevertheless, her physician daughter had encouraged her to continue trying and to enter rehabilitation programmes. These efforts had only yielded partial success. After the transfer to the nursing home, Mother's condition had deteriorated, perhaps due to new cerebrovascular incidents. Whatever the cause, ever since she had become less and less communicative. The fact that she began to dislike her daughters' visits was taken to be another signal that she felt abandoned in her requests to end her suffering.

The Postma doctors discussed the case at length and decided to end Mother's life. When they visited the nursing home that October day, they found Mrs van Boven unconscious and tied up on a toilet chair. Her daughter tried to wake her up. Unable to do so, she kissed her mother and took the syringe from her purse. While Mr Postma was guarding the door of the room, Mrs Postma injected 200 mg of morphine intramuscularly. A few minutes later, they called in the nurse; together they moved Mrs van Boven to the bed.

When the nursing clinic physician arrived at the patient's room about an hour later, he found Mrs van Boven lying in bed, dead, in the company of her family members. The next day, he called the authorities and a legal investigation was initiated. The year was 1971.[1]

The Dutch euthanasia debate

Ever since the 1970s, euthanasia has been a topic of continuous debate in the Netherlands and elsewhere. This volume presents a detailed description of the debate as well as a critical analysis of the most salient aspects of euthanasia practice. We will argue that euthanasia should be understood within a historical context as a protest against medical power. Paradoxically, the final outcome appears to be an unprecedented increase in medical power. Criticized by society for holding dying patients hostage with medical technologies and drugs, thus precluding a good death, Dutch society has granted physicians the right to end patients' lives with medical means. Physicians have thus acquired a level of power that nobody in the Netherlands has, not even the state, for the death penalty has long been abolished.

Debates about euthanasia commonly start with a 'paradigmatic case' to illustrate the relevancy and plausibility of euthanasia. The popular and scientific literature abounds with such cases about patients with incurable metastatic cancer, suffering from unrelieved pain, living in inhumane conditions, begging for an end. However, as the debate has developed over time, more and more cases have surfaced that differ significantly from these paradigmatic cases, suggesting that euthanasia might also be justified in other conditions and circumstances. We will analyse the evolution of the euthanasia debate in the Netherlands because there are evident parallels between the dynamics and politics of the Dutch debate and similar debates elsewhere in the world. Indeed, the same paradoxes tend to surface. In this volume, we will focus on two of the most troublesome paradoxes.

The first paradox results from the dialectical relationship between the moral principle of respect for individual autonomy and the moral principle of beneficence, in particular relief of suffering, as the two major justifications of euthanasia. Although euthanasia is an ultimate effort to give the individual patient control over his dying, the debate appears to have resulted in an increase of medical power. Perhaps even more troublesome is the second paradox. It concerns the very goal of euthanasia, that is, to bring about a good death. Although euthanasia originally emerged from a strong commitment to foster a good death, we will argue that the Dutch preoccupation with euthanasia may have actually threatened the range of options for patients to die a good death.

Modern medicine has yielded extraordinary benefits for mankind, extending life considerably and improving its quality. Unfortunately, there is no escape from death and hence no escape from dying. For many, the dying process has remained a very difficult period of life, filled with pain and suffering. Indeed, for some the power of medicine to prolong life has meant a prolongation of this dying process. This is a vexing problem for patients and caregivers alike, indeed for all of society. This book at once acknowledges the problem and argues against euthanasia as the solution to the problem. It is both a plea for more humility on the part of physicians, for acceptance of the inevitable limitations to the power of medicine, and a plea for a greater investment in genuine medical care for dying patients, that is, in the art and science of palliative medicine.

Beginnings of the euthanasia movement

Approximately one year after Mrs van Boven had died at the hands of her physician daughter, Dr Postma, the national newspaper *De Telegraaf* revealed that a euthanasia case was being investigated by the legal authorities. Previously, physicians had confessed on television that they had occasionally practised euthanasia, but no legal action had ever been taken. The revelation about Dr Postma and the subsequent media attention sparked several developments. First, the inhabitants of Noordwolde started a movement to support the Postmas. They considered it unjust that their family physicians were now the sole focus of legal attention, whereas euthanasia was more widespread throughout the country. This local action attracted the interest of several other national newspapers and television channels. Notifications of support from all over the country poured into Noordwolde. Almost 30 physicians from the province of Friesland officially declared that they considered euthanasia an act of compassion and therefore did not reject it in the context of medical treatment. Likewise, Baptist ministers in the northern parts of the country declared their solidarity with the Postmas.

Second, a lively public debate started with medical, theological, legal and ethical experts addressing various aspects of the issue of euthanasia. In retrospect, it is clear that the concept of euthanasia used was ambiguous. Expressions like 'not prolonging life', 'hastening death', 'choosing death', 'not obstructing the dying process' and 'forgoing medical treatment' were all classified under the generic label of 'euthanasia'. At the same time, all experts emphasized that euthanasia in practice was much more prevalent than accounted for in the media. They argued that medical practice had changed. The transitional line between life and death had been obliterated by modern medicine. Medicine had become capable of prolonging the life of patients, keeping them alive beyond any reasonable state of existence. Consequently, many patients now end up existing in a kind of no man's land between living and not living. The fear of ending up in this no man's land had already been ingrained deeply in the mind of the Dutch public as a result of an earlier case.

In 1966, Mia Versluis, a 21-year-old sports instructor who was about to enter into marriage, had undergone cosmetic surgery on her heel bones. During the surgery she suffered cardiac and respiratory problems which were not properly managed by the anaesthesiologist. She never recovered from the narcosis. Severe and irreversible brain damage had occurred. She was placed on a ventilator. After five months, the treating physician proposed to the parents to disconnect the ventilator. However, this proposal was commonly interpreted as euthanasia and the parents refused.

More than five years after the tragic surgery, Mia died without medical interference.

The case had attracted a lot of media attention. It demonstrated to the public mind not only the unprecedented power of medicine but also the risks involved. The lingering death of Mia had made many people extremely anxious about medical interventions that could keep patients in a state between life and death. The death of Mia Versluis on 10 November 1971 occurred while the (not yet publicly known) legal examination of the Postma case by the Leeuwarden District Court was taking place.

The third sequel to the publicity around the Postma case was the establishment of several societies and associations acting as public interest fora and political pressure groups. In February 1973, the Dutch Society for Voluntary Euthanasia was founded. Its aims are twofold: to promote the social acceptance of voluntary euthanasia as well as the legalization of euthanasia. In the same month, the Foundation for Voluntary Euthanasia was established (it was dissolved in 1985). This foundation, initiated by a number of scholars, well-known lawyers and physicians, had a different purpose: within the context of the existing legislation to develop and propagate a living will for euthanasia.

As a result of these media events and subsequent developments, the issue of euthanasia had already been transformed from a medical-legal problem into a social problem and public topic even before the Leeuwarden District Court decided the Postma case. That decision was reached some 16 months after Mrs van Boven died.

The verdict

The hearing took place on 7 February 1973 and lasted seven hours. Two weeks later the District Court of Leeuwarden issued its verdict. Although relief of suffering of her mother was a legitimate objective, Dr Postma had not used other means available to accomplish this goal. Ending the patient's life by administering a lethal dose of morphine is illegal. Dr Postma was therefore found guilty. However, the court imposed a probationary sentence of one week's imprisonment only. The public impact of the verdict was tremendous. Not only was the sentence very mild, but it was also an indication that the views on euthanasia in society, law and medicine were changing. More importantly, it was the first specimen of jurisprudence that did not categorically exclude the possibility of legally sanctioned euthanasia.

In its verdict, the court had accepted a number of conditions formulated by the court's expert witness, physician Hielke Kijlstra, the Health Care

Inspector of Friesland. He had argued that it is 'generally accepted in the medical community' that in particular circumstances patients may receive drugs to relieve their suffering but with the risk that life will be shortened. In these circumstances it is also accepted that life-threatening conditions such as infections will not be treated. Kijlstra had listed five conditions:

1 The patient is incurable due to a disease or accident.
2 In the patient's experience, the physical or mental suffering is severe or unbearable.
3 The patient has expressed a wish (maybe even in advance and in written form) to end his life or to be put out of his misery.
4 The patient has entered or is about to enter the terminal phase.
5 The intervention is performed by a physician, i.e. the attending physician or a specialist, or in consultation with a physician.

The court underwrote Kijlstra's list but also stated that condition (4) was too restrictive. Often incurably ill patients are suffering severely yet are not in a terminal state; they can continue to live in this condition for years. Mrs van Boven was an example. The court stated that these patients should also be offered the kind of palliative medical care mentioned above.

Even though the court's deliberations seemed to pertain first and foremost to palliative end-of-life care rather than euthanasia proper, the verdict had at least two implications for the subsequent euthanasia debates. It confirmed that the medical community had accepted certain limits to life-supporting treatment (the verdict actually referred to 'the average physician in the Netherlands'). It also listed certain conditions in which the death of the patient may be acceptable. In doing so, the court set an example of judicial reasoning about requirements of due care that could be followed by future courts. The verdict thus implied that death in the context of medical treatment need not be accidental, and that in certain specified circumstances the patient's death may be justified. The door to euthanasia had been set ajar.

Expansion of the debate

In its verdict, the Leeuwarden Court had argued by analogy. The circumstances identified in the verdict applied to the acceptance of the patient's death in the course of medical treatment but not due to the treatment. At the time, this was generally classified as 'passive euthanasia'. The court then applied the same line of thinking to the case at hand, even though that case was one of 'active euthanasia'. The court's argumentative strategy mimicked a more widespread logic of thinking about euthanasia. The starting point was the conviction that 'passive euthanasia' is permissible in specific circumstances. The case of Mia Versluis had illustrated that medicine could prolong life for a long time, indeed for too long a time. In such circumstances medical interventions to treat life-threatening events or to technically sustain life should be discontinued in order to avoid prolongation of the dying process. Next, it was argued by many Dutch (as well as foreign) philosophers and theologians that there is no moral distinction between 'passive euthanasia' and 'active euthanasia'. Hence, the legal conditions that were formulated for 'passive euthanasia' could be applied to 'active euthanasia' as well.

For example, Leenen, a well-known professor of health law in Amsterdam, argued that the distinction between 'active euthanasia' and 'passive euthanasia' is irrelevant from the perspective of Dutch law.[2] Moreover, the alleged moral difference should be rejected as well since it could imply that the suffering of the patient is prolonged if 'passive euthanasia' is accepted while 'active euthanasia' is desirable. Muntendam, a professor of social medicine in Leiden and one of the first chairpersons of the Dutch Society for Voluntary Euthanasia, likewise rejected the distinction because both 'passive euthanasia' and 'active euthanasia' require a considered decision by a physician, and in both cases the underlying motive is the same (i.e. relief of suffering).[3]

According to Leenen and Muntendam, euthanasia is not only analogous to palliative care, but in some circumstances it would actually be the preferred option. If termination of treatment is morally the same as terminating the life of the patient, one should not risk prolonging the patient's dying by merely forgoing treatment. It would appear more compassionate both to forgo treatment and actively end the patient's life.

We thus find that the Leeuwarden Court's inclusion of exonerating circumstances applicable to 'passive euthanasia' in its verdict about a case of 'active euthanasia' supported and boosted the existing euthanasia debate in the Netherlands. Now that legally sanctioned euthanasia had become imaginable, much intellectual activity was concentrated on a more detailed specification of the various situations in which it could occur.

As mentioned, the flurry of books and articles in these early years often presented paradigmatic cases showing the plausibility and acceptability of euthanasia. These cases usually contained the following elements: a competent patient with cancer is in a stage where the disease has become incurable; multiple metastases have led to a deteriorating condition with unbearable suffering; the patient is now in a terminal phase and is requesting euthanasia; this request is voluntary and persistent. The physician, confronted with the request, has a dilemma: Either (s)he respects human life, does not actively intervene, and accepts that the patient's suffering continues; or (s)he respects the patient's wish and hastens the patient's death through active intervention.

If this case would still not convince euthanasia opponents, a slightly adjusted case would be advanced in which the physician has absolutely no means left to relieve the patient's suffering other than to respect the wish of the patient to end her life. In such an exceptional paradigmatic case, many participants to the debate tended to accept the possibility of euthanasia. Even those who did not advocate euthanasia, often agreed that in such extreme cases euthanasia can be morally excusable.[4]

However, the most striking aspect of the Dutch euthanasia debate is not these paradigmatic cases. Rather, it is their being dismissed again as soon as they have been proposed. Almost all of the allegedly relevant elements of these paradigmatic cases in time have been dismissed as being too restrictive or even irrelevant.[5] Consider the first report of the Health Council on euthanasia which was released in February 1973, two days after the verdict of the Leeuwarden Court in the Postma Case (although it had already been finished in October of the preceding year). It proposed the following definition of euthanasia: 'Euthanasia is an intentional act to shorten the life or an intentional omission to lengthen the life of an incurable patient in his or her own interest.' Note that no reference is made to the request of the patient. A few months later, the Executive Committee of the Royal Dutch Medical Association issued a position paper endorsing the above definition. Several ethicists (even if they did not support euthanasia, e.g. Beemer[6]) agreed that the distinction between voluntary and nonvoluntary euthanasia is not watertight and of secondary importance from a moral point of view. Of primary importance is whether life is bearable and tolerable. Euthanasia may be acceptable not only if there is a request of the patient, but also if the patient assents to the suggestion of others, and even if euthanasia is in the patient's interest according to the judgement of the physician.

In 1978, euthanasia entered the political scene. The majority of the political parties in the Lower House of Dutch Parliament invited the Minister of Health to establish a national committee to develop policies in the area of euthanasia. This committee was finally inaugurated in 1982. In its report from August 1985, the committee defined euthanasia as 'the intentional termination of the life of a person by someone other than that person, at the latter's request'.[7] The Committee explained that terms such as 'incurable disease', 'terminal illness' and 'unbearable suffering' were not included in the definition because those are conditions under which euthanasia might be justifiable, rather than defining elements of the practice itself. Nevertheless, the exclusion of all these terms from the definition, versus the inclusion of the patient's own request, changed the euthanasia debate. The new definition became authoritative, often cited as the 'official' definition of euthanasia in the Netherlands, and the patient's request became the decisive condition. Euthanasia is justified if, and only if, it happens at the patient's explicit and persistent request.

However, in the late 1980s, it became evident that Dutch euthanasia practice did not conform to this official position. Many cases of euthanasia turned out not to involve an explicit request of the patient. But Dutch society, including the medical profession and the courts, did not rally against these cases. Instead, a series of new reports was issued by the Royal Dutch Medical Association examining the feasibility of euthanasia on several categories of incompetent patients. In the meantime, the courts imposed only suspended sentences for physicians who had ended patients' lives without their request.

In the 1990s, the movement towards decriminalization of euthanasia gained momentum. The labour, liberal and social-democratic parties combined acquired a parliamentary majority and the Christian Democratic Party was excluded from the government. A new bill to legalize euthanasia was submitted. The bill reiterated some of the old conditions such as the unbearableness of the patient's suffering and an explicit patient request. But as parliament was debating the new bill, two new cases underscored yet again that even these two conditions had long lost their decisive force.

The first involved Senator Brongersma, formerly a member of the Upper House of Parliament. He was 86 years old, had no physical or mental ailments, but was tired of living. In his view, life had become unbearable and an unacceptable source of suffering. Euthanasia protagonists argued yet again that this was the proper motive for euthanasia. After all, only the person himself can determine whether his suffering has become unbearable – even if the source of the suffering is life itself.

And then came the case of Van Oijen, the general practitioner who had figured prominently in *Death on Request*, the well-known television euthanasia documentary about himself. He was on trial because he had terminated the life of a nursing home patient at the request of the family rather than the patient. Van Oijen was found guilty of murder but not punished because he had acted 'with integrity' according to the court.

Thus we find that at the dawn of the twenty-first century none of the original elements that characterized the paradigmatic euthanasia case had survived. There was no need for a competent patient with incurable cancer; for multiple metastases causing unbearable pain; for the end of life to be nearing anyway; for an explicit and persistent patient request. Even though Dutch physicians were evidently euthanizing all kinds of patients who did not fit the paradigmatic case, in November 2000 the new bill was accepted by the Lower House of Dutch Parliament and in April 2001 by the Upper House. Euthanasia and Physician Assistance in Suicide had become legal.

The lack of a theoretical foundation for euthanasia

How can we explain these recurrent changes in the criteria for and justifications of euthanasia? We contend that a persuasive and resilient theoretical defence of euthanasia is lacking. Consider again the official Dutch definition of euthanasia that also underlies the new law: 'The intentional termination of the life of a person by someone other than that person, at the latter's request.' This definition suggests that the justification of euthanasia is grounded theoretically in the moral principle of respect for the autonomy of the individual patient. Although individual freedom is not as decisive a political principle as it is in the USA, Dutch people harbour strong libertarian sentiments that favour an almost absolute patient's right to respect of his or her autonomy. Consequently, in public debates on euthanasia it is generally taken for granted that the principle of respect for patient autonomy provides the necessary moral underpinning of euthanasia.

Yet on closer inspection, it is all but clear that the concept of patient autonomy can ethically justify the practice of euthanasia. Proponents of euthanasia have argued that autonomy implies the possibility and justifiability of making decisions about one's own death. However, this proposition is at odds with the philosophical and political tradition out of which the notion of respect for individual autonomy arose. In this libertarian tradition, autonomy has been deemed a basic characteristic of human beings because it guarantees that each person is free and able to make decisions according to his own free will. But the tradition has itself questioned whether an appeal to individual autonomy can ever justify ending one's own life. If autonomy is a basic value, can a person ever eliminate the very basis of this important characteristic? In order to be free, one has to exist at least.

This is by no means the only theoretical inconsistency. Even if one agrees that individual autonomy is a basic value, evidently it is not the only significant moral value. Consider the value of human life. Human life is of value not simply and merely because it enables autonomous decision making. Rather, human life is valuable even if persons do not or cannot make autonomous decisions. Newborns and children cannot make autonomous decisions, but their lives are obviously of great value. Indeed, much of human life defies the autonomy of the individual. The fact that we are born was not the result of our own autonomous decisions, nor the time and place of our birth, and neither is our gender, race, nationality and socio-cultural background. Moreover, much of what we have become is not the result of our earlier decisions. We are continuously confronted with conditions beyond our control, not because our autonomy is weak but because it is limited by the heteronomous conditions of life, many of which demand our respect. The first basic question in the moral debate concerning euthanasia therefore concerns the limits of autonomy.

If we were simply to assume that autonomous individuals have the right to end their lives, immediately another question emerges: Is it morally justifiable for other people to assist in this? Even if suicide is morally justifiable, that does not mean assisting in suicide is too. By definition, assisting in someone else's suicide is not an act that only concerns one's own life. Nevertheless, in the Netherlands it is generally assumed that assistance in suicide is justifiable if it is done by a physician. But why a physician? Again this is not self-evident because in other domains of life we actually prohibit physicians to end the lives of other people. Although the Netherlands does not have the death penalty, almost everybody agrees that of all people physicians should not be engaged in capital punishment.

Now even if we grant that the moral principle of autonomy justifies suicide, and that physicians may assist in suicide if so requested by the patient, it only follows that the doctor may prescribe the drugs necessary for the patient to end his own life. In order for the patient to execute his own autonomy, he must take final responsibility for his actions and end life himself by consuming the lethal drugs provided. But in euthanasia, it is the physician who administers the drugs and hence bears the final responsibility. This is clearly at odds with the primacy of the patient's autonomy. Nevertheless, assisted suicide has remained relatively infrequent in the Netherlands with euthanasia being almost ten times as prevalent.

The fact that euthanasia finally emerged as the primary and legal response to years of criticism against the power of active, interventionist medicine is ironic. From all alternatives explored in other countries, such as palliative care, hospices and forgoing treatment, euthanasia has turned out to be preferable precisely because it is a medical intervention: Not only a decision that is the prerogative of the physician, but also an act, the ultimate medical act in the face of death. We must thus conclude that respect for patient autonomy is a rather dubious theoretical justification for the practice of euthanasia by physicians.

Dutch euthanasia as a contradiction of respect for patient autonomy

To make matters worse, euthanasia not only lacks a persuasive and resilient theoretical foundation, hinging as it does on the principle of respect for patient autonomy. The Dutch practice of euthanasia also appears to contradict the primacy of the principle of autonomy. Research data in 1995 show that in comparison to an earlier study from 1990, the number of requests for euthanasia has grown.[8] A distinction is made between two types of patient requests. The first is a request to have euthanasia 'in due course'. For example, when patients are first diagnosed with cancer, many want to find out about their physician's stance towards euthanasia and they do so by asking for euthanasia. In 1995, more than 34,000 patients made this type of request (compared to 25,100 in 1990). Such requests do not necessarily mean that these patients want to die. They are anxious and afraid that the doctor, in a later stage when they will be suffering, will not do his or her utmost to relieve that suffering. A request for euthanasia is quite an effective way to assure the complete attention of health-care professionals. Indeed, many patients do not persist in their wish for euthanasia. In 1995, there were 9700 requests for euthanasia 'in the foreseeable future' (compared to 8900 in 1990). This second type of request for euthanasia typically occurs when the patient is at the final stages of her illness and death is imminent. The request forces upon the attending physician the decision whether or not to grant it. In 1995, of those 9700 requests 3200 were granted (compared to 2300 in 1990).

From these research data a striking conclusion can be drawn: Only a minority of explicit and persistent euthanasia requests is actually carried out. Two-thirds of the requests for euthanasia are not granted. Apparently the patient's own explicit and persistent request is not decisive. This conclusion is supported by other data, collected by the same research team. In 1995, Dutch physicians decided approximately 27,000 times to intentionally hasten the patient's death (whether by assisting in suicide, injecting lethal drugs, or withdrawing life-sustaining treatment). In approximately 60 per cent of these cases, this was done with the patient's consent. But the remaining 40 per cent occurred without such an informed consent.

These findings raise serious doubts about the significance of the respect for autonomy argument within the practice of medicine.[9] It appears that for medical doctors, respect for autonomy is not the decisive justification for action. In daily practice, the most important consideration and the main moral justification for euthanasia is relief of suffering. It is not really relevant whether the patients request euthanasia or not. If in the physician's opinion, patients are not suffering unbearably or their suffering can be treated, their request for euthanasia will not be granted. If, on the other hand, the doctor estimates that the situation of unbearable suffering is worse than being dead, (s)he will consider the option of active termination of treatment. In such dire circumstances, the patient's request to end life will support the decision, but it is neither a sufficient nor necessary condition. The empirical data reveal that many physicians simply assume that patients would have wanted euthanasia, even if patients have not been very articulate in requesting euthanasia or have merely hinted at the possibility of euthanasia, as well as if the patients are incompetent, psychiatric patients, demented elderly, or handicapped newborns.

These facts raise questions about the real justification for euthanasia. It is evident that from a historical perspective patient autonomy never figured prominently in the euthanasia debate.[10] Euthanasia was always considered first and foremost a form of 'mercy killing', an act of compassion where killing the person is better than letting him suffer. The history of the euthanasia movement in the USA shows that for a long time euthanasia was not primarily framed in terms of a personal decision or a merciful act, but rather as a public health measure. Euthanasia was justified because it was promoting the common good. It was in the interest of society or the human race, and removing burdens on society.[11]

In the present Dutch debate, both respect for patient autonomy and relief of suffering remain operative as justifications for euthanasia, even though it is theoretically difficult to combine the two and in practice they are often mutually exclusive. This paradoxical situation persists because consistency, that is, relying *either* on respect for patient autonomy *or* on relief of suffering, would yield unacceptable outcomes. For example, if autonomy would be truly decisive, ending human life without an explicit request would have to be ruled out. On the other hand, all serious patient requests for euthanasia would have to be granted. The number of euthanasia cases would be at least three times the present number. Very stringent rules and guidelines would have to be put in place to make sure that the patients' requests are reliable (e.g. repeated request, second opinion, documentation, etc.). But the grounds for the request can no longer be evaluated; they are the proper domain of the individual patient's valuation.

All of this appears quite consistent, but as the recent case of Mr Brongersma shows, the consequences of this logic are troublesome. If a patient, or rather, if a person claims that life itself is a source of unbearable suffering, one cannot argue against this claim. Nevertheless, in December 2002 the Supreme Court of the Netherlands rejected this line of reasoning. Concerned about the ever-increasing expansion of the euthanasia practice that looms when patient autonomy is the sole decisive criterion and justification for euthanasia, the court insisted that there must be some kind of medical condition explaining the suffering of the patient. But this shifts the discretionary power back to the physician, who has to independently assess the patient's claim of unbearable suffering. Only if there is a sufficient medical explanation for that claim can it be accepted and the request for euthanasia granted. In fact, it doesn't really matter whether the patient claims she is suffering unbearably. For even if the patient does not claim to be suffering (for example, because she is unable to do so due to advanced dementia), the physician can independently assess the patient's suffering. Now the question arises as to what the objective criteria are that allow a physician to judge whether the patient's suffering is unbearable indeed. Without such criteria, decision making will depend on the subjective and arbitrary values of individual physicians.[12]

Euthanasia as hindrance to a good death

The absence of a persuasive and resilient theoretical foundation for the practice of euthanasia has resulted in the gradual growth of medical power and the expansion of the euthanasia practice to ever more patient categories that have little or no resemblance to the original paradigmatic cases. In and of itself this is sufficient ground for serious concern. To make matters worse

– for patients that is – the Dutch developments may actually have decreased instead of increased their chances for a genuinely 'good' death.

The large-scale government supported empirical studies on Dutch euthanasia from 1990, 1995 and 2001 (the results of which will be discussed in more detail in Chapter 3), expectedly show that 'unbearable suffering' is most frequently mentioned by the surveyed physicians as reason for committing euthanasia. Next in line are 'dehumanizing condition', 'loss of dignity' and 'pain'. Considerably more surprising is a cluster of reasons that concern the individual patient's ability to cope with the situation: 'meaningless suffering', 'dependency' and 'tired of life'. These reflect the expansion of suffering as a justification for euthanasia from the somatic suffering of the paradigmatic cancer patient to mental and even spiritual suffering. Most remarkable is a third category of reasons that include 'escape from deterioration of suffering', 'prevention of suffocation' and 'prevention of pain'. These reasons show that euthanasia is no longer considered a way out of a state of unbearable suffering only, but also a sensible strategy to *prevent* such a state from occurring in the first place. Why wait until the suffering is becoming unbearable? The popularity of this new approach to euthanasia is evidenced by the fact that the former Dutch Health Minister herself suggested during the parliamentary debates on euthanasia that it would be wise for people in the early stages of dementia to draft an advance directive requesting euthanasia. She also advocated the distribution of suicide pills among the elderly.

The question arises whether the Dutch focus on euthanasia, emerging as an option in the search for a good death, has not at the same time reduced the range of care options available at the end of life. If euthanasia is no longer the option of last resort when all alternatives to relieve suffering have failed; if euthanasia instead has become a means of preventing such suffering altogether, there is no longer a need for alternative means of pain relief. Why develop therapies to mitigate patients' pain and suffering when euthanasia can prevent the emergence of severe suffering altogether? Why should society create social structures and networks to involve the elderly in human interaction and social life when euthanasia is an adequate remedy for older persons such as Senator Brongersma who experience loss of meaning in life? We thus find that the emphasis on euthanasia tends to deflect attention from other approaches to good death and dying.

Unfortunately, there is also empirical evidence to support this deflection. For example, many hospitals in the Netherlands only recently developed policies for withholding and withdrawing treatment. Expert centres in pain control and management have been established only in the last decade. Contrary to other countries, palliative care became a target of Dutch health policy only a few years ago.[13] Only now, after euthanasia has become prevalent and a legalized practice in the Netherlands, has a move towards the development of a wider range of available options at the end of life materialized, so that perhaps many requests for euthanasia can be prevented. Most recently, terminal sedation has become a trendy topic, which is a remarkable fact because it had always been discarded as a morally muddled approach, a concealed form of euthanasia and inconsistent with the principle of autonomy.[14]

These new developments are of course laudable but it may be a case of too little too late. Paradoxically, the commitment to a good death created the euthanasia movement; in turn the commitment to euthanasia reduced the number of options available to patients to bring about a good death.

A framework of queries

The Dutch experience with euthanasia is a social experiment that should be examined and scrutinized carefully by all protagonists as well as antagonists of euthanasia, both in the Netherlands and abroad. The experiment shows that the practice of euthanasia is paradoxical. Four fundamental questions must be raised and addressed:

1 Is euthanasia an appropriate answer to the problem of 'good death'? Those who answer negatively must show the superiority of other less controversial alternatives, but those who answer affirmatively still face other urgent questions.
2 If euthanasia is to be accepted: (a) what is the proper moral justification for this practice; (b) how can we prevent the dialectic expansion of acceptable cases?
3 If relief of suffering is the decisive justification for euthanasia: (a) how can we curb the impact of physicians' subjective judgements; (b) how can we make sure that physicians will explore, develop and apply alternative medical approaches such as palliative care?
4 If on the other hand personal autonomy is the decisive justification, how can this be reconciled with the fact that in euthanasia it is the *physician* who brings about the patient's death, thereby taking over the final and full responsibility from the patient?

Unfortunately, notwithstanding three decades of debate on euthanasia, these questions have yet to be answered in a clear, convincing and decisive manner. This book is an attempt to do so. To that avail, we will undertake a retrospective reconstruction in which we identify the main moral dimensions of euthanasia. This should enable a better insight into the development of the Dutch debate on euthanasia and the peculiar direction it has taken. We will find that the power of medicine defies social control and conclude that euthanasia is particularly difficult to manage and regulate from a policy perspective.

Some of the problems that Dutch policymakers face are related to the peculiarities of the Dutch legal system and to cultural idiosyncracies. Still, there is much to be learned from the Dutch experiment for any country considering regulating or legalizing euthanasia and assisted suicide. After all, the Dutch experiment has been very lengthy, spanning more than three decades and involving many possible regulatory systems (e.g. the medical profession, the health inspection, patient advocacy associations, disciplinary courts, criminal courts and the legislature). All of these systems have time and again failed and continue to fail, as we will show.

Indeed, there are many countries that may want to learn from this experiment. Consider the results of a 2003 survey by the Council of Europe on laws and practices concerning euthanasia and assisted suicide in 34 of its member countries and in the United States.[15] The first remarkable finding is the diversity in definitions across nations and cultures. For example, the distinction between 'active euthanasia' and 'passive euthanasia' is rejected in the Netherlands but used in 16 European countries. Almost no country has defined 'euthanasia' in its code of law. Notable exceptions are Georgia, which in its 1997 Health Law explicitly prohibits euthanasia, and Belgium, which in its 2002 Law on Euthanasia explicitly permits it. It is not even clear what it means to 'legalize' euthanasia, for according to the survey euthanasia is legal only in Belgium (and assisted suicide in Estonia and Switzerland). The Netherlands according to the survey has *not* legalized these practices. So how is it possible that Belgium, which based its law from 2002 on the new Dutch law, claims it has legalized euthanasia, yet the Dutch government in responding to this survey insists it has not?

Given that euthanasia is illegal in all other countries, how can it be explained that in only eight countries physicians have been prosecuted after performing euthanasia? Even in the 1980s when euthanasia was clearly illegal in the Netherlands, there were more than 100 cases on average each year. Thus, it seems highly unlikely that euthanasia never occurs in the other 26 surveyed countries. Whether or not it is practised, euthanasia has definitely become a topic of intense public debate in many countries. In addition to the Netherlands, Italy and the United Kingdom have had a national commission on euthanasia. In many countries, public bodies such as national bioethics commissions or parliamentary committees have issued regulations and recommendations. The need for some forms of regulation is increasing in many countries.

Finally, the Dutch experience shows that developments do not stop with legalization. Although one of the aims of the new law was to make doctors feel more comfortable in reporting euthanasia, the number of cases being reported is actually decreasing (from a high of 2216 in 1999 to 2054 in 2001), and this trend appears to continue after enactment of the law (1882 in 2002). Initially, it was hypothesized that this reporting decrease signified a decrease in the actual number of euthanasia cases allegedly due to improvements in palliative medicine, precluding the need for euthanasia.

But the latest empirical report by Van der Wal and colleagues proves otherwise. The number of euthanasia and PAS cases continues to rise (from 3600 in 1995 to 3800 in 2001).[16] This would suggest that the new law is failing to achieve its main objective, that is, increased reporting and hence increased quality control.

Since the enactment of the new euthanasia law, remarkable positive developments have occurred as well. The general practitioners who in years past had been trained to become a national network of euthanasia consultants are now also trained in palliative care so that they are able to suggests alternatives to euthanasia. The number of hospices, palliative care units and palliative care consultations teams has significantly expanded over the last few years. Although the overall and long-term significance of these recent developments cannot be assessed at this early time, it appears that the legalization of euthanasia has led to a certain pacification of the debate, creating room for alternatives, palliative approaches and strategies to prevent euthanasia. A new image of death and dying is emerging – 'palliated death'.

2 The growth of medical power

Victims of medical power

'Human life may be ended by the physician. In two ways. By discontinuing medical treatment, and by performing a medical act. In the first case, the physician is passive ... In the second case, the physician is active. He kills the patient.'[17] With this conclusion Van den Berg summarizes his monograph *Medical Power and Medical Ethics*. The publication rapidly gains acclaim as well as notoriety, resulting in a request by several Dutch Members of Parliament to the Minister of Health to establish a committee that will study the problem of medical power and medical ethics. In turn, the Minister asks the Health Council for advice regarding the apparent and increasing uncertainty about medical-ethical issues in the country. The Council's Ad Hoc Committee publishes its interim advice on euthanasia in 1972. The euthanasia debate has begun.

Jan Hendrik van den Berg was a psychiatrist and professor in the Faculty of Psychology at the University of Leiden. Educated in phenomenological approaches (the subject of his doctoral dissertation), he was inclined to give priority to observation and understanding rather than theory and abstract models. From a phenomenological perspective, reality is not an inventory of exact and unchangeable components and data. In his *Metabletica*, Van den Berg developed a doctrine of changes and changeableness ('metabletica' is derived from the Greek *metaballein*: changing, transforming).[13] Instead of describing continuities, he sought to identify moments of innovation and discontinuity. No innovation, not even a scientific development, can be understood when dissociated from the changing context of cultural patterns.

Van den Berg's metabletic theory is akin to, but developed independently of the theories of the American philosopher of science Thomas Kuhn (1922–1996) who published *The Structure of Scientific Revolutions* in 1962, introducing the notion of a 'paradigm' to explain the nature of scientific change. Metabletics is also related to the ideas of the French philosopher Michel Foucault (1926–1984) who distinguished (especially in *Les mots et les choses*, 1966) epistemological structures or 'epistèmè' that typify the discontinuous development of history.

Characteristic of Van den Berg's theory is his insistence that the external world presents itself to us in two different aspects, each with its own reality. In its first structure, the reality of the external world has an authentic existence with changeable manifestations and meanings. In its second structure, the reality of the external world is stable and unchanging and of human-made character. The objects in the second structure are quantifiable, measurable and immutable, and therefore the focus of the scientific perspective. However, in their first structure, objects transcend the fixed framework of measurable quantities. They have discontinuity. They are evolving, transforming and continuously self-projecting. This first structure is uncovered when we adopt a phenomenological rather than scientific perspective that focuses on the meaning and interrelatedness of objects.

Van den Berg considers this phenomenological perspective generally to be of more significance than the scientific perspective. In *The Human Body*, he outlines how the scientific perspective on the human body has changed time and again in the course of history under the influence of scholars like Vesalius and Harvey. Van den Berg shows that the anatomical body is really an abstract and a derivative of the living body projected into the realm of death. Rather than the corpse, the living body is far more interesting and significant. It has meaning and is creating meaning in the complexities of real daily life and in the interconnections with the transforming culture in which it exists.[19]

Because of the mistaken belief on the part of modern medicine that the scientific perspective and the quantifiable reality have primacy, modern medicine is at an impasse when confronted with ill and dying patients. This mistake is Van den Berg's motive for writing his book on the human body. In it he presents a case of a 70-year-old patient, diagnosed with renal cancer, but refusing treatment and hospitalization. He discusses the resulting quandary for the family physician who wants to treat the patient. The physician is trained to fight disease, to cure, to act because he wants to rescue and prolong human life. He views himself as the enemy of death, the protector of the body. But against which death should he fight? Is the physician also the enemy of the death that is desired by the patient? Is the physician also the protector of the living body that longs for its expiration?

Van den Berg points out that the family physician could have found support in the Hippocratic Oath which emphasizes the interest of the patient, giving priority to the ill person over the disease. In *The Art*, another work attributed to Hippocrates, medicine's three goals are defined: (1) to take away the complaints of ill persons; (2) to relieve the intensity of their suffering; but also (3) to abstain from treatment when the patient's illness is incurable. This third goal has almost been forgotten in modern medicine. The basic fact that all human beings are mortal and, hence, fundamentally incurable is neglected in present-day medical science. The Hippocratic lesson is that it can never be the duty of physicians to cure all people all the time. For every patient, the doctor must reflect on the balance between the powers of the disease and the powers of the ill person.

The same ideas are reiterated and specified ten years later in Van den Berg's publication on medical ethics. Although the number of pages is insignificant compared to the earlier works, this small monograph had a far greater impact, not in the least because of the dramatic examples included. The monograph starts with a case about a child with spina bifida. In the five years of his life, the child has had six surgeries and an enormous number of complications. In retrospect, the boy's life can be considered one long road of suffering. It can also be regarded as the triumphal march of medicine that succeeded in overcoming most setbacks and emergencies. The case demonstrates medicine's newly gained power. But the nature of this power is primarily technical. It is grounded in advances of microbiology, medicine's success in treating and preventing infectious diseases, the development of surgery and transplantation, resuscitation technology and the production of effective drugs.

Paradoxically, medicine's new power has made the basic principle of medical ethics obsolete. Since the beginnings of medicine, this principle has demanded that the physician should preserve, rescue and prolong human life at all times. The doctor should be the ally of life, the enemy of death. But this principle is fundamental only as long as the physician has little power. Precisely because he had little to offer, the physician was urged to utilize all available means. But now that medicine has become extremely effective, it is no longer clear that the doctor should always intervene.

Van den Berg underlines this thesis with several examples. He presents a photograph of a hydrocephalic patient and questions the treatment decisions that have prevented the patient from dying. The monograph also includes a picture of a child with phocomelia due to the use of thalidomide. Van den Berg comments that giving these children a lethal injection is 'an act of simple, medical devotion to duty'. Medical power should be used to end a human life when medicine itself has seriously damaged that life. One of the most dramatic photographs shows a patient with hemicorporectomy: the whole lower half of the body has been removed surgically. Whereas the authors of the *Surgery* article in which the case was described originally call it 'a successful lumbo-sacral operation', Van den Berg characterizes it as 'a medical-ethical offence'.[20]

Van den Berg believes that these instances of overtreatment are in part the result of medicine's failure to involve the patient. The patient should determine whether medical treatment should be carried out. At any moment, the patient should be allowed to refuse continuation of treatment. This freedom of the patient arises necessarily out of the very power of modern medicine. The physician deceives himself when he thinks that he is the authority, the expert who provides assistance and even cure. In the face of technology, physician and patient are equal. Sooner or later, they will have to communicate, deliberate and share in the decision-making process. The application of technical power demands non-authoritarian communication. The physician who wants to use this power must first talk with the patient about illness and approaching death. In doing so, he cannot force the patient to adopt his own scientific perspective on the human body. Physician as well as patient must be able to freely choose between a body in the first or in the second structure of reality.

Van den Berg continues his discourse with examples of patients who are unable to decide for themselves. For instance, the parents of a comatose patient with irreversible brain damage decide that she should be given a lethal injection. While granting that at present this is not legally possible and that most doctors will refuse, Van den Berg forecasts: 'But it will happen. It also should happen.'[21]

Medical-ethical uncertainty

Van den Berg's publication is a rhetorical but vigorous argument for a change in attitudes: More and better communication with patients, more patient influence in decision making, increasing attention to illness and dying. These issues all gained prominence in the bioethics movement of the last quarter of the twentieth century. However, his book also propagates a new ethic: Medicine should continue to preserve, rescue and prolong human life if and where it is meaningful; but it should also intervene to terminate life that is damaged, handicapped, disfigured, decaying, and has lost its dignity and meaning. Van den Berg grants that it is difficult to demarcate meaningful from non-meaningful life. He suggests that a committee consisting of several physicians and lay members must make decisions regarding the death of patients. But regardless the committee's decision, Van den Berg insist that the patient himself should determine how he wants to be ill, and how he wants to die. As long as the patient persists in expressing his wishes, the physician shall follow.

Van den Berg's publication had a significant impact. In just a few years it had been reprinted more than 20 times. Member of Parliament Dirk Willem Tilanus Jr (1910–1996), a family practitioner and the spokesperson of the Christelijk-Historische Unie (CHU), a political movement that existed from 1908 to 1980 and consisted primarily of members belonging to the

Reformed Church, referred to the increasing uncertainty in matters of medical ethics. He argued that the progress in medicine had evoked many ethical and existential quandaries concerning artificial insemination, contraception, abortion, euthanasia, determination of death. These quandaries had created fundamental uncertainty among physicians. He believed it was important that the physician 'adapt himself to modern society and make himself familiar with modern thinking of people'.[22] Tilanus therefore submitted a request to the Minister of Health to establish a committee to study the problem of medical power and medical ethics.

Minister Roelof Kruisinga, who also was a physician and a member of the CHU, responded by asking advice from the Health Council of the Netherlands. The council had been established in 1902 as a permanent professional advisory body, advising the government on the advancements in scientific knowledge about health care and the environment.[23] Until the 1960s, ethical issues played a minor role in the council's reports. Minister Kruisinga was the first to explicitly demand an ethical analysis. In response, the president of the Health Council inaugurated an Ad Hoc Committee on Medical Ethics, composed of 16 members (physicians, lawyers, nurses, ethicists and sociologists). In 1977, a Standing Committee on Medical Ethics and Health Law would be established.[24]

The newly established Ad Hoc Committee struggled with the Minister's broad advisory request: 'Is it from the perspective of medical ethics allowed for the physician to use, not to use, or no longer use available medical-technical and pharmacological possibilities in order to bring into existence human life, independent or not, or not to create human life, ending it, or lengthen the process of dying?' The Committee decided to focus on the topic of euthanasia 'because it seems to be most urgent'.[25] At the same time, it observed that the ethics of the medical profession was in flux. Norms that had been generally accepted in earlier days were no longer widely endorsed. But a new and uniform perspective on medical-ethical norms remained lacking. Instead, a plurality of continuously changing viewpoints had developed. For this reason the committee deemed it difficult to outline generally accepted moral rules. The committee therefore decided to publish an interim advice only.

Normative stability

The predicament of uncertainty in medical ethics, pointed out by Tilanus and the Health Council's Ad Hoc Committee, was a new experience. Medical ethics, as in most other countries, had always been the prerogative of the medical profession. In 1936, the Royal Dutch Medical Association had published the first edition of its *Medische ethiek*. The book is an overview of the duties of a physician, concentrating on 'the leading principles', and written 'to the benefit of the medical profession in The Netherlands'.[26] It perfectly illustrates an understanding of medical ethics as 'deontology', a code of conduct which consists partly of moral rules, partly of rules of etiquette, and partly of rules of professional conduct. This conception assumes that only a good person can be a good physician. A physician should have many virtues in order to maintain the continuous trust of patients as well as society at large. At the same time, the reader will look in vain for an explication of medical-ethical principles. It is obvious that principles are implicitly accepted. A good example is the instruction about informing patients. This should always be done such that the patient's hope of recovery is maintained. The justification for this instruction is both brief and simple: 'The physician has the task to defend life, to be the advocate of that life.'[27]

The authors of the handbook could afford to be so brief because their advice was reflecting moral convictions common at the time. For example, in his 1929 book *De ethica aan het ziekbed* (Ethics at the bedside), retired hospital director Wortman stresses the significance of giving courage to patients. In turn, he quotes the famous nineteenth-century German surgeon Theodore Billroth's claim that hope is the best medicine to relieve suffering because man lives by hope. The primary duty of the physician is to provide the patient with all the pleasure and energy of life possible until the natural end of life, as if all organs are functioning normally.

Wortman also discusses euthanasia, but this term is used in the literal and traditional sense of the word as the condition in which life comes to an end calmly and quietly. The task of the physician is to make this process as easy as possible, depriving death from its image of terror and attenuating its bitterness. The author raises the question whether it is allowed to intentionally shorten a life that is coming to an end. The answer is a short and pertinent 'no'. Regardless of how much the physician is moved by compassion or pressured by the patient or his relatives, it is never permissible to accomplish an easy death at the expense of life.

The postwar period

The Royal Dutch Medical Association published the second edition of its book on medical ethics in 1941 but did not revise it 'due to the current circumstances'. However, the changes in professional practice and the increasing interaction between medicine and society in the 1950s necessitated a revision. The third edition, published in 1959, shows at least two significant changes. First, the authors point out that the traditional understanding of medical ethics is ambiguous at best; it appears to include both moral rules and rules of conduct and etiquette. The title of the book has therefore been expanded into *Medische ethiek en gedragsleer* (Medical ethics and instructions on conduct) to underscore the distinction between the two. The authors furthermore explain that medical ethics is more than professional ethics; it cannot be based solely on the internal morality of medical practice. The foundations of medical ethics are in fact not different from those that underlie all human activities: 'Medical ethics is ethics in medical matters.'[28] This explanation reveals that a very new concept of ethics is developing. The values, norms and rules prevailing in social, cultural and religious traditions that function as external determinants of medicine (the 'external morality') are gradually gaining more weight and relevancy in medical ethics.

The second change concerns the principle of respect for human life. Whereas this was implicit in the first edition, now it is made explicit. The basic task of the physician is to help a human being in need, especially when human existence itself is threatened. Hence, the primary duty of a physician is the fight to maintain the patient's life. As stated by the World Medical Association, this fight should be fought so as to maintain the utmost respect for human life. According to the Royal Dutch Medical Association, this implies that the medical professional must always strive to preserve life. This is a demanding task. For example, the physician may not omit efforts to maintain life because he assumes that further efforts would only increase the suffering of the patient. Furthermore, it is argued that the physician may not cooperate with, or even passively observe, a patient who is trying to kill himself. It is the duty of the physician to protect the patient against himself. But the physician's task is also limited. After all, 'it is precisely not the task of the doctor to pass a judgement on the meaning of suffering or the meaning of existence itself, neither in general nor in relation to the significance it can have for the person of the patient.'[29] Here we find the stringent scientific perspective that Van den Berg will later criticize as one-sided. The value-laden phenomenological reality is considered outside the scope of appropriate professional medical care.

The authors of the third edition acknowledge that the physician must also relieve suffering, even if it implies some risk to the patient's life. Although they do not invoke the doctrine of double effect (about which more will be said in Chapter 5), the model is clearly applied. For example, it is never allowed to intentionally shorten the life of a suffering patient, even if this is done to limit the suffering. This maxim reflects the second condition of the model which states that the bad effect (the patient's death) may never be the means to achieve the good effect (relief of suffering). Furthermore, the physician should seriously consider the potential dangers to the patient's life when applying efforts to relieve suffering. This maxim reflects the fourth condition that there must be strong reasons to tolerate the bad effect (the patient's death) when pursuing the good effect (relief of suffering).

The authors also recognize that problems will arise when the patient himself objects to continuation of life and declines the care offered by his doctor in an attempt to hasten his death. Such a refusal will be more acceptable to the physician if he agrees that there is no hope for the future of the patient. But even if there is still hope, it is not justified to force the patient into accepting unwanted medical treatment. The physician will have to resort to persuasion for he is neither the master of the patient nor his servant. Again, the views of the Royal Dutch Medical Association as expressed in the third edition of the handbook are in accordance with the generally accepted moral convictions of the time. A good example is the 1948 book *Arts en patient* (Physician and patient) by surgeon Dr Salomon, written for medical students and young physicians. In his view, medicine is applied humanism; ethics is the mother of medicine. Especially now that all moral values are disgraced, it is necessary to revitalize ethics. Following Albert Schweitzer, he presents respect for life as the basic principle of ethics: 'Good is: to maintain and protect life; bad is: to destroy and damage life. The ethically minded human being does not ask whether this or that life is of any value; life in itself is sacred for him.'[30]

A survivor of the war, Salomon's concerns are clearly motivated by the horrendous lessons learned from World War II. Confidence in the medical profession had been shaken severely by the atrocities revealed during the Nuremberg trials in 1945 and 1946. Medical organizations discerned an urgent need to explicate the norms of medical ethics and specifically to underline the principle of respect for human life. The experiences of World War II also instigated international cooperation. In 1947, physicians from 27 countries founded the World Medical Association (WMA), an international, independent confederation of professional medical associations. It was created to ensure the independence of physicians and to strive for the highest possible standards of ethical behaviour and care. During its second General Assembly in 1948, the WMA adopted the Declaration of Geneva as its answer to the shocking engagement of German physicians in the Nazi programme for the destruction of 'lives not worth living'.

The 'mercy death' programme of the Nazi regime had killed over 70,000 patients, not only incurably sick, but also psychiatric patients, the mentally handicapped, and deformed children. The programme was designed to rid Germany of its weak, handicapped and 'inferior' citizens. The underlying philosophy was crude: patients were to be either cured or killed. The extermination, euphemistically labelled *Sterbehilfe* or 'assistance in dying' was carried out in special euthanasia institutes (*Euthanasieanstalte*) at the initiative and with almost full cooperation of the medical profession. Doctors were neither obliged nor ordered to kill psychiatric patients and handicapped children. As Proctor states: 'They were *empowered* to do so, and fulfilled their task without protest, often on their own initiative.'[31] If there were complaints, they focused primarily on the fact that the operation was not legal, because it was not legitimized by a euthanasia law. Although proposals for such a law were widely discussed, none was ever formally adopted by the Nazi government. In response to public criticism, in August 1941 the regulated programme (with registration, medical observation and deportation to special institutes) was stopped. But so-called 'wild euthanasia' – as Menges calls it[32] – continued: every physician could kill patients as he deemed appropriate, though the methods (starvation, intoxication) were less conspicuous than before. The policy decision was to regard euthanasia as a private matter, an issue to be dealt with in the relationship between physician and patient. Menges estimates that the total number of victims of the various euthanasia activities in Germany between 1939 and 1945 exceeded 100,000.

The 1948 WMA Declaration of Geneva (which has since been amended several times, most recently in Stockholm in 1994) contains a loud and clear rejection of any activities by physicians akin to those committed in the context of the German euthanasia programmes. This declaration is actually a rewrite of the Hippocratic Oath in view of modern developments. It is a secular oath in which physicians, at the time of being admitted to the medical profession, pledge to consecrate their lives to the service of humanity and to practise medicine with conscience and dignity; that the health of the patient will be their first consideration, and that they will maintain utmost respect for human life. The WMA recommends the new oath to medical schools and practising physicians because it endorses fundamental principles of medical ethics which can be applied to the current circumstances of health care regardless of cultural and religious traditions.

A year later, at the third General Assembly in 1949 in London, the International Code of Medical Ethics was adopted (and revised in 1968 and 1983). It summarized the most important principles and reformulated these as duties. For example, a physician shall in all types of medical practice be dedicated to providing competent medical service in full technical and moral independence, with compassion and respect for human dignity. Under 'Duties of Physicians to the Sick', it is stated: 'A physician shall always bear in mind the obligation of preserving human life.'[33] In 1964, the WMA adopted the Declaration of Helsinki which covers the ethical principles for biomedical research with human beings as they were developed initially in the context of the Nuremberg trials. This code of research ethics has been amended several times, most recently in Edinburgh in 2000.

One of the remarkable characteristics of these early codes and declarations is the absence of any rights language. The Declaration of Geneva is phrased in the traditional first-person language of the earliest moral documents in medicine, starting with the Hippocratic Oath. The International Code is phrased in terms of rules and duties. Veatch has speculated that the Nazi experience may have fostered the language of rules rather than rights.[34] But even these rules are written from the perspective of the physician rather than the patient who can lay certain claims. The final foundation for the norms specified is still the internal morality of medical practice. The core principle calls for the physician to do what he thinks will benefit the sick. It is simply assumed that only doctors can determine what is needed in any given case.

The changing medical scene

Postwar medical science advanced more rapidly than ever before. Its diagnostic potential and therapeutic effectiveness progressed steadily and significantly. Most physicians vested strong confidence in science and cherished optimistic expectations about the power of future medicine. They had no doubts whatsoever about the scientific character and methods of their profession.

There were some, however, who were less assured. Medicine itself became an object of reflection. The distinction between the science and the art of medicine was articulated. A debate ensued as to whether medical science was too much focused on studying and treating specific components and functions of the diseased organism (the hallmark of medical specialties) rather than treating the patient as a whole person (the hallmark of general practice). A 1959 editorial in the *Nederlands Tijdschrift voor Geneeskunde* (Dutch Journal of Medicine) signals the roller-coaster of contemporary scientific and technical innovation but also points to the difficulties in applying the theoretical knowledge in daily practice. Excitement over advances is concomitant with concern over possibilities for control.

Scientific and technological advances

For the purposes of this book, the debate about resuscitation technology is of particular relevance. The technique of external cardio-respiratory resuscitation had just been described in the literature, as well as the artificial ventilation technology and the first intensive care units. The many ethical problems that will later surface on the agenda of the bioethics movement are already identified in this early stage. Critics point out that resuscitation prolongs the dying and intensifies the suffering of the patient; death is postponed yet a cure is out of the question. The use of newly developed technologies creates ethical problems when the obligation to respect life is interpreted as an absolute principle. An ever more widespread concern arises that modern medicine, notwithstanding the best of intentions, will bring about situations that are unbearable and unacceptable. Writing in a 1959 issue of *Medisch Contact*, the journal of the Royal Dutch Medical Association, Kooyman points out that technical medicine confronts us with questions about the meaning of existence, about the nature and purpose of disease and suffering.

The discussion in the medical journals of the time also shows that ethical concerns notwithstanding, these new technologies are eagerly welcomed and quickly accepted as ordinary means of intervention. Resuscitation technology is applied as long as the nature and extent of the underlying medical condition is not clarified. Artificial ventilation is readily used. Once started, most doctors are unwilling to discontinue ventilation. Instead they prefer to wait until complications arise and then no longer treat these. A 1960 survey reveals that approximately half of the responding Dutch physicians will continue with ventilation until the death of the patient.[35]

The old rule *in dubio abstine* (when in doubt, abstain) appears to have been replaced by a new rule, more compatible with the new technologies: If there is doubt, act. As long as there is still a chance of recovery, the physician must apply life-saving technology. Galbraith has called this the 'no lose philosophy' in medicine.[36] It not only reflects a particular pro-life ethos but also a specific method of decision making. This method rests on the presupposition that disease or abnormality are present unless proven otherwise. It is better to presuppose the existence of a pathological process while in fact nothing is wrong, than to overlook an actual process. False-positive findings are less serious than false-negative ones.

These ethical and methodological underpinnings of the unrestrained adoption of new technologies in medicine's arsenal cannot prevent that by the late 1960s, uneasiness was spreading within the profession itself. Whereas most physicians had been deeply involved in or at least impressed by the revolutionary progress of medical science, now an increasing number among them were calling for a new critical and ethical awareness. In 1966 Thung questioned the self-assurance of medical science. Physicians should not simply assume that the goals of the new medicine are worthwhile and meaningful. Not all progress can be interpreted as a genuine improvement. Medicine must acknowledge its limits.

Thung is not alone in his criticism. Leading professors of medicine are raising questions about the advances of medical science. In connection with the development of organ transplantation, Orie questions whether the evolution of medicine these days is really a rational affair. In view of the rapid advances, there is a serious need to reformulate the goals of health care.[37] Den Otter is even more critical than Orie. He complains about the frightening influence of medicine on contemporary society. If we want to exert any influence on the way scientific medicine evolves, we need philosophy and religion as guides. Like Orie, Den Otter believes that the primary target of these moderating and directing influences shall be the personality of the doctor. He does not believe these disciplines shall or can affect the process of scientific inquiry or the factual content of scientific statements. The contribution of philosophy and religion is primarily in the field of ethics where they can foster the wisdom and moral qualities of the clinician.[38]

Orie and Den Otter recognized the need for reflection on the applications and social consequences of medical knowledge, and on the responsibility of the individual physician for the immediate and remote effects of his actions. This attitude towards philosophy characterizes the medical profession in the late 1960s. It makes clear why and to what purpose, in 1968 a philosopher was asked to contribute a paper for a leading Dutch medical journal. Although limited in its scope, Van Peursen's discussion of the consequences of recent advances of medicine for the patient, the physician and the community, is a genuine novelty. It is also a sign that the very progress of medicine itself had caused the domain of medical ethics no longer to be the exclusive territory of physicians.

Anthropological medicine

The growing influence of philosophy in medicine is also apparent in a movement that was most important in Germany but quite influential in the Netherlands as well. The 1950s and 1960s were the heyday of so-called anthropological medicine. Here, the term 'anthropology' refers to the philosophical subdiscipline that studies humanness. Thus, anthropological medicine is medical theory and practice that is specifically informed by such philosophical reflections on the nature of being human.

The leading Dutch representative of this movement was Frederik Buytendijk (1887–1974), the central figure of the Utrecht school of scientists employing the phenomenological method in medicine, psychology and pedagogy. This school also influenced Van den Berg in his early academic career in psychiatry. Many proponents of anthropologically oriented medicine are practising physicians and prolific writers with a broad interest in the humanities. Their main interest is to redefine and reinterpret medicine as a science of man. In philosophically rethinking medical activities, they use ideas from several contemporary philosophical schools, particularly phenomenology (Husserl, Merleau-Ponty), existentialism (Marcel, Sartre), and philosophical anthropology (Scheler, Gehlen, Plessner). They reflect on human existence in its concrete specificity and ambiguity. Instead of starting from or working towards an ideal image of the human being, they attempt to identify what is anthropologically characteristic and common to human beings. But at the same time they are very much aware that any image is too abstract and clean. For in everyday reality the specific individual is always changing, multiform, and not fully described by the designed image of human being.

One basic tenet in the anthropological tradition is the rejection of Cartesian dualism.[39] Human beings cannot be subdivided into physical and mental compartments. Although medicine has profited from this subdivision, it has also restricted itself to the human body, studying and explaining the body's physical-chemical machinery. This medical approach to the human being and its body is problematic because it reduces the human being to an animal species, and the human characteristics of the human body to its physical level of being. Dualistic thinking not only involves a reduced image of the human person, but it is also reductionistic in a more general sense, as evidenced by the distinction commonly made between object and subject. The leading German proponent of anthropological medicine, von Weizsäcker, strongly rejects the idea that there is an objective and real world, independent from an isolated and individual subject. Conversely, a human being cannot relate him/herself to the world as an neutral observer. We can only know the world in which we live by living in it and hence changing it at the same time.[40]

A second tenet is that medicine should be regarded as the science of the human person. Anthropologically oriented physicians argue that the methodology of the natural sciences is not fully appropriate in the context of health care. Scientific methods are abstract and analytical, assuming a model of linear causality. These methods also focus on intervention, control and manipulation, introducing the technical point of view that is characteristic of the engineer into the domain of disease and suffering. Note that causal thinking and the technical approach of the natural sciences are not rejected outright. On the contrary, their value and usefulness are readily acknowledged. But medical thinking and practising should not restrict itself to these scientific methods. These methods have only relative value for medicine, for they can never grasp the essence of being human. The abstract and analytical methodology of the sciences necessarily disconnects and disintegrates the unity that characterizes the patient as living organism, as person. Once one adopts the mechanical viewpoint of the scientific method, the only characteristics of living organisms that can still be explained are those that are not intrinsic to life itself.[41] Anatomical, physiological and biochemical research only determines the conditions; they teach us what is possible and probable, but never what really happens. The macroscopic images of bodily events, the dynamic Gestalt, and the intrinsically meaningful connections have disappeared from the scientific view.[42]

The third basic tenet of the anthropological movement is its insistence on the need for a comprehensive understanding of disease. According to anthropologically oriented physicians, the prevailing conception of disease is incomplete. The reason is not that the science of pathology is insufficient or not yet fully developed, but that pathology operates with inadequate notions and assumptions. When focusing on the causal mechanism of disease, medicine cannot fully understand the ill person. In order to truly explain disease, one must gain insight into the significance of the symptoms, which in turn requires that the meaning of a particular complaint is addressed.

The proponents of anthropological medicine insist that disease always has meaning. The body gives expression to the human person. Being ill is a way of being a human person. I not only *have* my body; I always *am* my body as well. Hence, I never only *have* a disease or suffer it passively as something that overcomes me. I always *am* my disease as well and hence make my disease. Being ill is a response of the person to his or her own individual existence. From this perspective, disease is never merely blind fate, an objectionable event waiting to be eliminated from the world. The important thing is what we make of it, whether we consider it as an occasion to reconsider and improve our lives.

Although the influence of anthropological medicine quickly waned by the end of the 1960s, it paved the way for and thus fostered the emerging interest in medical ethics since the 1960s. It did so by criticizing the presuppositions of the dominant conception of medicine as natural science, and by incorporating the analytical methods of medical science and its mechanistic image of the human being into a much broader framework of an authentic science of the human being. The programmatic demand of von Weizsäcker to introduce the subject into medicine implied not only an acknowledgement of the subjectivity of the knowing and acting subject (the physician), but also that of the object (i.e. the person passively undergoing the medical activities). Consequently, in order to fully understand diseases, the physician must always consider the personal biography of the patient. The scientific perspective tends to orient the physician upon organic life (*zooè*) rather than upon biographical life (*bios*). This perspective is important for a correct understanding of health and disease, life and death. But for a correct understanding of the patient's own experiences in undergoing the disease as well as the therapy mounted in response, the physician must gain insight into the life world of the patient and the biography of the person.

The debate about general practice versus specialization

The twentieth century has been called 'the age of specialization'. The major specialties of medicine emerged, and they soon differentiated into super-specialties. Medicine's shift from extramural primary care to intramural specialty care is exemplified in the rapid growth of the number of hospital beds in the Netherlands from 36,000 beds in 1945 to 58,000 in 1960, and to 72,000 in 1970. Medical education likewise took a disease- and specialty-centred turn. General practice was surpassed by intramural health care both technologically and quantitatively. Whereas specialists had been unknown in the beginning of the twentieth century, by 1970 they outnumbered general practitioners.[43] Because of the revolutionary progress of specialized and hospital-based medicine, the position of the general practitioner became increasingly problematic. To make matters worse, the number of physicians available for primary care declined, even though the total number of physicians increased from 0.63 physicians per 1000 inhabitants in 1940 to 1.31 physicians in 1972. Hence, the number of patients per general practice multiplied.

The crisis in general practice during the 1950s and 1960s was urgent because general practitioners continued to hold a key position in the Dutch health-care system. By 1964, Dutch general practitioners had 60 million patient encounters annually and they treated 90 per cent of all patient complaints.[44] But the pressure exerted on them revealed the need to examine their own discipline. General practitioners began to ask what 'general practice' really means. What distinguishes it from medical specialties? What is its essence, its identity, its character? The Dutch equivalent of the 'general practitioner' is the *huisarts* which literally means 'house physician'. This connotation of housebound medicine is lost in both the British term 'general practitioner' and the American 'family physician'. But precisely this connotation was the starting point for a debate on the new tasks of the general practitioner in the era of medical power.

The process of reflection was started by Buma with his book *De huisarts en zijn patient* (The general practitioner and his patient) from 1950. Buma delineates the field of activity as well as the tasks of the family doctor. He raises the question: What should one know to call oneself a general practitioner? This question implies a critical examination of the foundations of medical theory and practice. Buma criticizes the almost exclusively scientific nature of these foundations. The experiences of the general practitioner underscore that anthropological problems are as important as medical problems. In addition to his analytical schooling and scientific way of thinking, a general practitioner needs a comprehensive view and a personal approach. For the general practitioner, human understanding is often more important than causal explanations of disease mechanisms. Buma concludes that general practice urgently needs an anthropological foundation; the next phase in the evolution of medical science should be anthropological medicine.

There was a second reason to re-examine and redefine the nature of general practice. The patients' problems were changing. Instead of acute illnesses, ever more patients presented themselves to the general practitioner with chronic ailments and psychosocial complaints. A new kind of generalist was needed, with a patient-centred method and a different, more holistic scope. General practice should embody a new paradigm in which the whole person is the focus of concern and care rather than organs and diseases. General practice should make the task of the physician more comprehensive: 'To understand the physical nature of the illness but also to understand the patient and the meaning the illness has for him or her.'[45]

These theoretical deliberations found a practical effect in 1956 when the

Nederlands Huisartsen Genootschap (Dutch College of General Practitioners) was founded as the professional organization of general practitioners. A special conference proposed to define general practice as family medicine, and gave a now well-known description of the function of the family doctor: to accept responsibility for a continuous, comprehensive and personal care of the health of all individuals and families who have entrusted themselves to him. In 1958, a professional journal was started (*Huisarts en Wetenschap*). The first chair in family medicine was established in 1967; ten years later all eight medical schools had departments, educational programmes and chairs in this area.

The reawakening of general practice was associated with the unease regarding the new technological and scientific possibilities as well as the anthropological criticism of medicine. The emphasis on the doctor–patient relationship, the fact that every Dutch citizen has a general practitioner, that the general practitioner gives continuous care (sometimes even a lifetime) as well as personal care (meeting patients in his office or in their home), and his role of gatekeeping (guiding referrals to specialists) have all been articulated at some point as characteristics that can control the negative impact of technical medicine. Given these characteristics, it is at least understandable why general practitioners were the first to protect their patients against medical activism and interventionism.[46] Because of their longstanding relationship with their patients, family practitioners believed euthanasia ought to be the prerogative of physicians.

Medicine's social status

During the 1950s and 1960s the Netherlands, like other European countries, created a complicated welfare system. Health care, social policy and legislation became interwoven through several important laws. In 1964 the Social Health Insurance Act was passed. Two-thirds of the Dutch population were now covered by social health insurance through the sickness funds (statutory below a certain income). This created a social security health insurance system in which employee and employer both pay part of the premium. The remaining one-third are insured by means of private health insurance or civil servant health insurance.

Two major principles were underlying this policy: (a) Equal access to health care for all citizens, and (b) solidarity between the poor and the rich, the sick and the healthy, and the young and the old. The same principles guided the Exceptional Medical Expenses Act (AWBZ) from 1967. This law addresses long-term care or other treatments that carry a prohibitive price tag, such as specialized services for mentally or physically handicapped, psychiatric care, and home nursing. It created a compulsory health insurance scheme in which everyone between 15 and 65 years of age must pay a compulsory premium, levied together with income tax. Income loss due to illness or disability is covered by other types of insurance. About the same time that these laws were passed, health-care costs began to rise dramatically from 3.3 per cent of the GNP in 1953 to 6.3 per cent in 1970, increasing even further the influence of policymakers on the provision of health care. But the medical profession itself also became more and more involved in the implementation of social policies. In 1959, social medicine was recognized as a separate medical discipline and medical specialty.

But the optimism and enthusiasm about the progress of medicine and the welfare state were not unconditional. Publicity about several very serious medical mishaps dampened the excitement. The first was the thalidomide drama. The impact was more strongly felt in Europe than in the United States. Thalidomide was developed and first marketed in West Germany. It was prescribed from 1957 as a sleeping pill. At one point more than one million Germans used the drug every day. Adverse effects (such as neuritis) occurred but initially were not reported. The situation drastically changed when in 1961 the first cases were reported of rare and gross foetal deformities (phocomelia) when the drug was used by pregnant women. The total incidence of the birth malformation induced by the drug was over 8000 in 46 countries combined. The event aroused great public concern. It created worries about careless science, unreliable information and unwarranted prescribing.[47] The drama led to more and better regulations and drug control, demanding pre-marketing testing with respect to efficacy and safety. But it also stimulated the uneasy feeling that increasing medical power could produce conditions that were no longer 'humane'.

Widely publicized was the court case in the Belgium city of Liège in November 1962. The parents of a baby seriously handicapped due to thalidomide had killed their child after consultation with the family physician. The jury acquitted the parents. Public opinion as well as printed media were squarely in favour of the parents. As we have seen earlier, the case of the thalidomide child was also used by Van den Berg in his critique of the power of medicine and the pro-life emphasis of the prevailing medical ethic.

The second dramatic event was the case of Mia Versluis (summarized in Chapter 1). For more than five years she was in a vegetative state due to a medical accident during anaesthesia. The case received enormous public attention. There was frequent talk about 'euthanasia' in the subsequent discussions because the anaesthetist had proposed to the father to discontinue the ventilation. Nowadays, the court's use of the term 'euthanasia' to characterize the anaesthetist's proposal would be incorrect. But in the late 1960s, the concepts of euthanasia versus forgoing treatment had not yet been clearly demarcated. The latter was commonly considered to be 'passive euthanasia' and hence a form of euthanasia. More remarkable than the use of the label 'euthanasia' was the court's reasoning. The court noted that in 1966 (when the anaesthetist's proposal was made) the views regarding intervention in the dying process were even less clearly articulated than at the present moment (i.e. in 1969). Hence, the physician was not to blame. Only the way in which the proposal had been made (without preceding consultation with a colleague) was blameworthy.[48]

Thus a paradoxical situation emerged. There was widespread public excitement about new medical interventions and a shared willingness to make all of these resources available for all citizens through a comprehensive health-care system. All of this boosted the status and power of the medical establishment exponentially. But there was also a growing suspicion about all of the alleged medical progress, fuelled by mass media reporting on some of medicine's most dire mishaps. Public ambiguity spearheaded debates about the adverse effects of medical power and the need for a new medical ethics.

Secularization

Before we examine the results of these new debates about medical power and medical ethics, one more social development must be reviewed because it is of particular relevance for a proper understanding of the development of the euthanasia debate, that is, the religious situation in the Netherlands. One of the most salient features of Dutch society is the rapid process of secularization, especially between 1965 and 1975. In 1960, 37 per cent of the Dutch population were Catholic, 28 per cent Dutch Reformed, 10 per cent neo-Calvinist, and 21 per cent regarded themselves as non-church members. The Catholics and neo-Calvinist were very lively religious communities at the time, having their own systems of schools, hospitals and mass media. Felling and his colleagues observed that in comparison with other west and north European countries, the Netherlands was a genuinely devout nation in those days.[49]

In the relatively short period between the second half of the 1960s and the end of the 1970s, drastic changes occurred. Religious beliefs, church involvement and the importance of religion in daily life all became less important. The Catholic part of the population was mostly affected. The large and powerful Catholic network of social institutions and organizations was rapidly dismantled. Catholic intellectuals disseminated new ideas promoting tolerance, freedom of individual conscience in ethical issues, and integration of Catholics into Dutch society. Church leadership was exceptionally permissive.

By international standards, the beliefs of the Dutch today are very secular; church membership is extremely low compared to other countries. For example, in 1987 the percentage of the population affiliated to any church was 94 per cent in the USA, 91 per cent in Austria, 76 per cent in the

United Kingdom and a mere 46 per cent in the Netherlands.[50] By 1996, only a minority was still a member of an established church (21 per cent Catholic, 14 per cent Dutch Reformed and 8 per cent neo-Calvinist).[51]

The period during which the euthanasia debate emerged is therefore characterized by an enormous decline in church orthodoxy. These developments were leading to a rapid transformation from a religious into a secular nation. A 1981 comparative survey in nine European countries demonstrated that the Dutch are much more permissive on moral issues than the other countries.[52] Catholics hold much more liberal views on moral matters than members of other denominations. For example, a survey in 1996 showed that only 8 per cent of Catholics were opposed to euthanasia, compared to 32 per cent of Dutch Reformed and 36 per cent of neo-Calvinists.[53] This rapid transformation makes Dutch society a prime example of the process of secularization.[54] In the Christian tradition, existential crises in human life such as suffering and dying could be interpreted in a framework of transcendent meaning. Since human life is sacred and inviolable, it must be respected. Ultimately, decisions about life and death are not ours, precluding abortion, euthanasia and suicide. But such interpretations are not compatible with a secular world view. The idea of an untouchable natural order is rejected. Increasing significance is given to the conscience of the individuals who distance themselves from the authority of the church and religion. Doctrinal truths no longer have relevance for daily life. Instead, the humanistic view gains prominence that life and death are natural phenomena whose meaning is created by humans. Each individual must shape this meaning by interpreting life's events according to his or her own values.

As a result of this process of secularization, sociologists have concluded that the Netherlands is no longer a Christian nation. It has shed its identity. The traditional religious nature that was once a vital characteristic of the Dutch is today only a characteristic of certain subgroups.[55] It is not easily explained why these changes occurred so rapidly and intensively. The most usual explanation assumes that the secular climate in the Netherlands is a reaction to the rigidity of the earlier compartmentalization of society along denominational lines.[56]

The power of medicine

Given the advances of science and technology, the anthropological reorientation of medicine, the revival of general practice, and the intertwining of social legislation and health care, we can better understand why Van den Berg critiqued the recent and unprecedented power of medicine, and why his critique was well received at the time. As was also argued by proponents of anthropological medicine and protagonists of a new type of generalist physician, there was the danger that medicine through its new scientific and technological capacities could easily interfere with human interests and transgress the boundaries of meaningful life. Van den Berg argued that this new power required a new medical ethic as a counterbalance. Some acts of today's powerful physicians are objectionable from a moral point of view, although they were mandatory in the deontology of an earlier powerless medicine. Though Van den Berg's concrete suggestions for a new ethic (e.g. active euthanasia of defective newborns) caused controversy inside and outside the health-care professions, his monograph was an eye-opener to many, and made clear at once the need for renewed medical ethics. His monograph showed that medical power should be contained, and in some circumstances resisted. One of the counteracting measures could be euthanasia.

An interesting draft for a new ethical approach was made by Paul Sporken (1927–1992), a Roman Catholic priest appointed in 1974 to be the first holder of the first chair of medical ethics in the Netherlands at the University of Maastricht. His book *Voorlopige diagnose* (Provisional diagnosis) was published in 1969, almost at the same time as Van den Berg's monograph. Sporken's book was the first synopsis of a medical ethics that departed from traditional deontology. He did not base his medical ethics on absolute moral criteria for medical practice but took his starting point at the patient–doctor relationship. Ethics requires a continuously developing understanding of what it means to be an authentic human being. Moral judgements must be anchored in our image of human beings and human dignity. Sporken also discussed the problems of end of life care. Aiding the dying patient (*stervenshulp*) is a medical-ethical duty. It implies the creation of optimal conditions for the patient 'to die his own death'. Abandoning the patient in the terminal phase is therefore out of the question, but it remains controversial how assistance should be provided. Sporken concludes that a categorical prohibition of euthanasia is untenable if (and only if) the patient himself has decided that his life is completed. Euthanasia is therefore morally acceptable in exceptional circumstances.

In the 1972 edition of his book, Sporken discusses the ideas of Van den Berg. He agrees with most of these ideas but strongly emphasizes the autonomy and real interests of the patient as the basic norms of medicine. He disagrees with Van den Berg's conclusion that in some cases it is not only the right but also the duty of the physician to kill the patient. Sporken first objects that there are no criteria to determine whether the life of a patient must be considered meaningless, especially in the case of handicapped children. His second objection concerns the input of the patient in the decision making: Euthanasia without the knowledge and will of the patient is wrong. Sporken acknowledges that sometimes the prolongation of life no longer has meaning; medical power then dehumanizes the patient. But it is incorrect to conclude that termination of life is acceptable in these cases. The correct conclusion must be that such interventions should never have happened, or should be discontinued. If we can no longer assist life, we should assist in dying. But this is not the same as active euthanasia. Euthanasia in these circumstances is a symptom of impatience to let the patient die his own death. In other words, it does not respect the person of the patient, but constitutes the physician's flight from his own incapacity to accept the limits to his medical power.

In his discussions about the relationship between medical power and euthanasia, Sporken refers to debates about the proper role of medicine as well as medical power. These debates as they have developed since the early 1970s can be broken down into three subsequent phases, each of which has also impacted the euthanasia debate. During the initial phase, medical power and its consequences are first recognized and criticized. The work of Van den Berg has been conducive in raising the issue of euthanasia in this context.

The next phase is characterized by intense critique of medical power. The notion of 'profession' is used in a pejorative sense and even interpreted as 'stronghold of wiseacres'.[57] The rapid growth of medical power is a sign that medicine has totalitarian inclinations. It should therefore be confined within clearly marked boundaries, and the effectiveness of medical knowledge even within these boundaries is doubted. Dutch editions of the books of Illich (1975) and Zola (1973) became popular and were often quoted. Even more influential was *De markt van welzijn en geluk* (The market of well-being and happiness), written by the Dutch philosopher Hans Achterhuis in 1980. He generalized the ideas of Illich, and claimed that they are relevant to all health professions, including social workers.

Following Zola,[58] these critics of the medicalization of society focused on medicine as a major institution of social control and blamed the medical profession for being largely responsible for the new burden of disease, for the increase of disabling dependence, or for undermining the ability of individuals to cope with illness and suffering.[59] The point is not only that medicine's effectiveness is often overestimated, but it is also harmful; so much so that the medical establishment has become a major threat to health. Illich introduced the notion of 'iatrogenesis' to label the disease, dysfunction, disability and pain that are the result of technical medical interventions. One more negative outcome of the growth of medical power is its penetration into daily life and ordinary experiences, transforming the usual meanings of these experiences. Pain, suffering and death are transformed into accidents for which people must seek medical treatment. Finally, the medicalization of social life and culture has an even more fundamental effect. It destroys 'the potential of people to deal with their human weakness, vulnerability and uniqueness in a personal and autonomous way'.[60] Because of medicine's alleged power, medical authority is allowed to intervene in the lives of people on behalf of their own health; it has made people dependent on the professional management of pain, sickness and death. Everything has been so arranged that people themselves lose their power and will for self-sufficiency; they finally 'cease to believe that autonomous action is feasible'.[61] This is particularly noticeable in the area of death and dying: 'The medicalization of society has brought the epoch of natural death to an end. Western man has lost the right to preside at the act of dying ... Technical death has won its victory over dying.'[62] This was the underlying fear of the euthanasia movement: the individual was completely alienated from his own death; the choreography of the dying process was fully in the hands of medical professionals.

The third phase in the debate on medical power is characterized by attempts to neutralize, pacify or reduce medical power. In this period it was repeatedly argued that the position of those who require care should be strengthened through democratization and emphasis on the rights of patients. Initially, the key word was *mondigheid* (assertive involvement). Medical power should be shared. The responsibility of the patients must be recognized. They should have a voice in the decisions that are made in regard to their own disease and suffering. From this perspective it is not permissible that physicians alone can make significant decisions that influence the lives of patients.[63] However, a new discourse soon developed that emphasized patient rights, self-determination and respect for patient autonomy.[64]

The debate about medical power demonstrates that several seemingly independent phenomena are actually connected. The advances of medical science and technology require an increasing specialization with a focus on hospitalization aimed at life-saving and curative interventions. This growth of medical power is associated with a growing dependency of people on medical professional management. This development in turn creates a climate of increasing unease about and dissatisfaction with dark sides of medical progress. In response, the need to foster generalist approaches and in particular to strengthen the position of the general practitioner is recognized, as well as the importance of patient input. Because medical power has expropriated the power of the individual to heal himself and to shape his environment, the balance must be redressed by giving more power to patients. If health, in the words of Illich, is 'the autonomous power to cope', recuperation of personal responsibility for health care must be the central issue.[65]

A new focus on death and dying

This is the context in which euthanasia surfaced as an issue of intensified debate. By the 1970s, mortality patterns had changed significantly. Two characteristics that had dominated human dying for the previous century had become much less important: acute death due to infectious diseases and childhood death. The new death that is most significant for modern man is associated with old age. The new dying is associated with chronic illness and hence protracted. Furthermore, death and dying were once social events in which the community was participating and supporting. Nowadays, death is a more private affair, of concern to family or the individual alone; death has disappeared from the public sphere and become less and less visible. Unless they are old, not many people are confronted with death and dying. At times, death is even denied by modern culture. For many people it is an abstract topic. Even for the elderly, acceptance of human mortality and finiteness is a difficult process.[66]

In 1969, Elisabeth Kübler-Ross published *On Death and Dying*. With narratives of the experiences of terminal patients, and with an analysis of the various phases of the dying process, Kübler-Ross put the topic of death and dying on the public agenda. She argued that emotional support and counselling in the final phases of human life are necessary interventions. The dying person should be allowed to die his or her own death. Because life and death are continuous, living is preparing oneself for death. The dying process, the very last stage of one's life, is life's fulfilment. A good death is not fundamentally different from a good life.

But the ethos of medical interventionism precludes the patience and tolerance required by the respect for the process of dying one's own death. The availability of medical services and the medicalization of society have reduced the capacity of individuals to care for themselves and to face suffering and death. Conversely, the medical profession has come to view death as the ultimate enemy. It is to be combated with all available means. Even the cultural image of death changes in the second half of the twentieth century.[67] The French historian Philippe Ariès (1914–1984) characterized this new image as 'forbidden death'. Death becomes 'wild', shameful, and it disappears from public life. This is due to a change in the place of death. People no longer die at home amidst relatives and family. The hospital is the place to die, often after a long medical struggle against death. Death is not an inevitable biological event with which the individual has to come to terms, but a medical failure or at least a topic of technical concern demanding constant involvement by medical professionals. Death is an unfortunate accident rather than a ceremonious ritual.[68]

In 1970, 56 per cent of Dutch people still died at home or in an elderly persons home, whereas almost 40 per cent died in hospital. But even dying at home no longer meant dying without medical care. In 1974 Van Es observed that in an average general practice (with 3000 patients), the general practitioner is confronted with 25 dying persons annually, most of whom he can supervise.[69] In other words, even if patients die at home, they need medical attendance and supervision. The trend towards hospitalized death in the Netherlands has since progressed. By 2002, only 30 per cent of all Dutch people still died at home (even though 75 per cent expressed the wish to die in their own house).[70]

In this context, the issue of euthanasia appears as an effective way of not only breaking the taboo of death but also countering the medical appropriation of death and dying. The euthanasia discourse brings together the two major critiques about death and dying. On the one hand there is the medical management of mortality; on the other hand we find the alienation and depersonalization of dying through technical interventions. In order to renew the image of and approach to death it should first of all be accepted that death is not a mere accident; it is the product or outcome of a long series of activities and interventions. Mortality is manageable and should be managed, but it should be the prerogative of the dying person himself rather than the treating, caring and supporting physician, let alone the medical profession. A new vocabulary reveals the shift in the locus of control: death at request, choosing death, right to die, desired death. The patient choreographs his own dying; he is the director of his final performance. But it is also a solo performance. Present-day citizens regard themselves first of all as autonomous individuals, as independent and thus isolated subjects. This is what the sociologist Elias has called the self-image of the 'homo clausus'.[71] We live alone and likewise we die alone. It is but another expression of the value of individual autonomy.

The new medicine can provide the possibilities to control death by empowering the individual to dispel death, fully and quickly. The victory over death, which was the aim of modern medicine, can finally be accomplished because it has become the aim of patients themselves; they want a fast, painless and regulated death, and medicine is the perfect instrument to arrange it. Indeed, according to professor of moral theology Kuitert, the physician must comply. He is obligated to grant a request for euthanasia. After all, it is the physician who prevents a gentle ending with his medical interventions. Medical progress has closed so many entrances for death into our lives that only the most bitter and miserable exits have remained. The same doctor who has rescued our life and has prolonged our life with his medical technologies should also procure a merciful death if we request him to help us.[72]

The new image of euthanasia as a medical as well as a personal achievement is exemplified in the television interview with Frans Swarttouw, a prominent Dutch businessman known as 'Mr Fokker' (after the aeroplane business he managed). The posthumous broadcast in February 1997 resembled a farewell interview. The master of industry, ill with cancer, announces his plan to 'die like a gentleman'. He wants to be master of his own fate. As one of the obituaries points out: 'He never delegated his power as director.' Dying itself is a manageable opportunity.

The same ideas have been elaborated more recently by Chabot, the psychiatrist who assisted in the suicide of a psychiatric patient in 1994. As the title *Sterfwerk* (Dying labour) indicates, Chabot considers dying a task, a 'job'. Suicide can be a dramatic composition (dramaturgy); it is the final act of the self with its personal *mise-en-scène*, perfectly prepared and staged, and completely different from the impulsive and desperate suicide. It is the ultimate presentation of self in death.[73]

Development of the practice of euthanasia

The initial and challenging defence of euthanasia in the monograph of Van den Berg was quickly followed by a much broader public debate on euthanasia. Even though little was known about existing euthanasia practice, public opinion polls showed an increasingly positive attitude towards active euthanasia (41 per cent in 1972; 59 per cent in 1983). The first study about euthanasia practices in Dutch hospitals was only published in 1983.[74] This study showed that many physicians and nurses are confronted with questions from patients about euthanasia. Forgoing life-sustaining treatment appears to be common, but there seems to be a lot of hesitation among health-care professionals about active euthanasia. In the same year, however, two general practitioners frankly admitted that they had performed active euthanasia on some patients, and they described their cases in medical journals.[75]

The public discussion about euthanasia was intensified after 1973. For the first time in Dutch history the District Court of Leeuwarden declared euthanasia acceptable under certain circumstances. A series of court decisions followed (analysed in Chapter 4) in which various legal strategies for getting around the existing criminal prohibition were tried. But by the early 1980s, outright legal forbearance was not yet politically acceptable. For example, the Dutch Catholic bishops launched a strong and well-argued protest against these legal developments. Apart from this protest, the political parties in parliament had only just begun to consider the issue. In 1983 a National Commission was installed to study the problem and to advise government about possible legalization of euthanasia.

In the meantime, many discussions on principles took place between moral philosophers, physicians, theologians and lawyers. Unfortunately, these debates were often confounded by the multiplicity of definitions for the term 'euthanasia'. According to Klijn and Nieboer, the term had actually lost its usefulness with respect to the subject concerned. It was used for too many practices, ranging from withdrawing life-sustaining treatment that has been refused by the patient to ending a patient's life without a request from the patient. By using a single term for a variety of practices that from an ethical and legal perspective are fundamentally distinct (see Chapter 5), these important differences were masked. Klijn and Nieboer also signalled the troublesome tendency in the Dutch debate to merge euthanasia and assistance in suicide, even though they are distinct legal entities in the Dutch Penal Code. In the case of euthanasia it is the physician (or another third person) who kills the patient. But when the physician assists in suicide, it is the patient who takes his own life. The physician merely assists in the process. This makes a real difference in responsibility. By overlooking these important distinctions, an undifferentiated and broad concept of ethical responsibility emerges in which the physician is always equally responsible for the death of a patient.[76]

The ethical debate concentrated on the distinction between forgoing life-prolonging treatment when there is no expectation of improvement (which was commonly mislabelled 'passive euthanasia'), and intervening in the patient's dying process at the latter's request in an explicit attempt to bring about her death ('active euthanasia'). Most ethicists and physicians considered forgoing treatment morally acceptable, provided the usual norms of careful decision making are abided by (e.g. the physician may not paternalistically override the will of the patient). Such forgoing of treatment is admissible when and because it only involves a judgement about the value of certain medical interventions, not about the value of the patient's life. Conversely, euthanasia proper involves a judgement about the value of the patient's life. It is at this point that the views of moral philosophers, lawyers, physicians and others diverged.

On one side of the debate authors such as Sporken and Dierick argued that distress, pain and suffering as such have no value; they are meaningless.[77] But it is not up to us to judge life itself as meaningless because of that distress. Each person is unique, irreplaceable and as such enjoys intrinsic dignity. This dignity is also inalienable. Neither others nor the person himself can abolish his own dignity. However, the meaningfulness or value of human life does not always coincide with the meaningfulness or value of medical treatments. When medical interventions have become meaningless because they cannot foster the patient's quality of life or even harm the patient, they may be forgone for exactly that reason.

The other side of the debate was represented by authors such as Leenen and Kuitert. In their view, the right to self-determination as such can ethically justify suicide, assistance in suicide as well as euthanasia proper.[78] Leenen's insistence that euthanasia must always be voluntary resulted in the Netherlands' officially adopting a definition of euthanasia that includes the condition 'at the patient's request'. Euthanasia by definition is voluntary. However, a fundamental question remains whether or not this right to self-determination is an absolute right that includes the right to end one's life. In the preamble and in Article 1 of the Universal Declaration of Human Rights, human freedom is based on the acknowledgement of the inherent dignity and the equal rights of all human beings. This suggests that the right to self-determination is not absolute but always secondary to the intrinsic dignity of the human person. Moreover, it is philosophically dubious that the right to self-determination can ever be invoked to justify a right to end one's own life, for the latter right would make all further exercise of the former right impossible.[79]

As if to strike a balance, Sporken argued that the concept and practice of euthanasia should be limited to the dying process, defined as the situation leading irrevocably and shortly to death. Furthermore, euthanasia ought to be an intrinsic element of the process of care of the dying. It should be an ultimate option, not a presupposed possibility.[80] However, Klijn and Nieboer objected that Sporken's limit to the practice of euthanasia would probably not hold because there are no fundamental reasons to abide by it. The limit is emotional only and hence will succumb.[81] The developments in the late 1980s and early 1990s would confirm their worry.

These fundamental ethical and legal tensions remained unresolved into the 1990s. But the stalemate did not stall the developments. If anything, they progressed ever more rapidly. Various attempts to legally regulate euthanasia were undertaken. Several large-scale empirical research studies were published. The practice of euthanasia even became television entertainment when the documentary 'Death on Request' was broadcast on Dutch television in October 1994 (as in various other countries thereafter). Euthanasia began to lose its restricted status as a rare and last resort escape from the ravages of terminal cancer. In its verdict of 21 June 1994 the Supreme Court concluded that the mental suffering of Dr Chabot's patient did not preclude assistance in her suicide. The state of suffering is more important than the existence of somatic illness or the terminal phase of an illness. What counts as unbearable suffering is in fact within the competency of the patient. This ruling caused upheaval because many doctors now felt that they could be requested to end the lives of patients with mental and existential problems. They feared medicine was becoming an instrument to end the life of a patient who does not want to live anymore, whatever the reasons. Psychiatrists in particular argued that it is wrong and dangerous to interpret the suicidal wishes of depressed patients as a genuine euthanasia request.

But then again, the importance of the patient's request as ardently advocated by early supporters of euthanasia such as Leenen was also diminishing. Government surveys from 1990 and 1995 disclosed that each year a considerable number of patients' lives were ended without the explicit request of patients themselves. But the data caused remarkably little outcry in the Netherlands. In fact, the number of proponents of legalized nonvoluntary termination of the life of an incompetent patient only seemed to increase. Professional committees established by the Royal Dutch Medical Association, the Dutch Society of Paediatricians, and the Dutch Society of Psychiatry agreed with the Supreme Court that psychiatric illness does not necessarily reduce the patient's voluntary decision-making competency; hence, the acceptability of euthanasia cannot be ruled out a priori.

But even if a patient is evidently incompetent (e.g. comatose or a disabled newborn), actively terminating the life of such a patient can be morally justifiable.[82]

In April 1995, the Court of Alkmaar was the first to consider a case of active termination of the life of a severely handicapped newborn. Dr Prins was exempted from punishment because the suffering of the neonate had been so severe that it provided a moral justification for ending her life; an additional justification was found in the parents' wishes that she die. This case was followed by another one later that year, in which Dr Kadijk gave a lethal injection to a baby with trisomy 12, a severe genetic abnormality. This physician was again found not liable to punishment because he had acted out of his medical-ethical duty to alleviate unbearable suffering.[83] Opinion polls showed that by the middle of the 1990s, public agreement with life termination without request was even more frequent than agreement with euthanasia (69 per cent versus 56 per cent).[84]

This development from voluntary to nonvoluntary termination of life had already been predicted by Theo Beemer in 1986: 'I am convinced that the criterion of voluntary request, formulated as a demarcation between morally acceptable and morally unacceptable killing, will not hold.'[85] Beemer, a Catholic moral philosopher, insisted that self-determination is not the only relevant ethical issue. Euthanasia is also always about mercy killing and compassion. He complained that the public debate was more or less pacified at the expense of suppressing and concealing half the story. However, this pacification strategy is in vain because this part of the story will time and again reappear, in medical practice, in journals, in ethics committees. This restriction of euthanasia to termination of life at the explicit request of the patient, as the official Dutch definition would have it, will not prevail. Indeed, the emphasis on a voluntary request causes all kinds of difficulties in the area of end-of-life care for neonates or incompetent patients. It results in the construct of the fictitious or presumed will. What would the person himself have willed if in this situation he had been able to express his will? This construct is dangerous, according to Beemer, since it obliterates the distinction between voluntary and nonvoluntary killing. The views of other people are easily projected onto the incompetent patient, as if the latter would have willed himself what reasonable third persons or common sense prescribe. The second difficulty with the criterion of voluntary request is that only the voluntariness of the request may be assessed, not the actual contents or the reasons behind the request. But Beemer pointed out that, quite inconsistently, many criteria had been formulated to defend and justify the request for euthanasia other than it being voluntary (such as 'last resort' or 'unbearable suffering'). Beemer's conclusion was that regulation of the euthanasia practice was 'half-hearted'; it had only focused on one part of the problem.

The issue of public control

Another development that has continued to provoke debate is the question of public control. How is review and evaluation of the euthanizing physician's justifications to be carried out? The recent law enacts a notification procedure (which actually had been operative for some years). However, the procedure appears to be rather ineffective. A substantial number of euthanasia cases (possibly as many as half) continue to go unreported. One of the main reasons for physicians not to report these cases is their dislike of the complex judicial procedure entailed by the notification procedure.[86] Physicians who do not report tend not to consult with a colleague either (as required by the official guidelines). In only 18 per cent of cases in which a physician did not report euthanasia is another colleague consulted. In cases of life termination without the explicit request of the patient it is a mere 3 per cent.

For several reasons it is doubtful whether the objective of better public control can be accomplished. First, society's possibilities for controlling the practice of euthanasia are entirely dependent upon the cooperation of those who are involved in this practice. Second, the new law is itself unusual. On the one hand, euthanasia has remained illegal even after the Criminal Code was changed in April 2002 for those physicians who do not abide by the formal requirements of due care; yet on the other hand, the same physicians are required to disclose their illegal conduct. It is paradoxical to require physicians to assist in their own arrests by disclosing their illegal actions, even more so when those actions legally constitute one of the most serious crimes (i.e. homicide). The law even provides physicians with official documents to be used when disclosing this crime.

This paradox aptly illustrates the ambiguous stance of the government (and society at large) towards euthanasia. On the one hand it considers killing human beings, though seriously ill and on the verge of death, an extremely problematic practice requiring legal restrictions and judicial audit. On the other hand, the government appears unwilling to rigorously scrutinize the medical profession. It sides with the profession's view that deviations from normal medical practice by individual physicians within the intimate doctor–patient relationship are simply a token of the physician's conscientious respect for the patient's personal wishes. In order to protect this mutual trust and respect between physician and patient, the privacy of their relationship may not be opened up to public scrutiny. If society grants physicians the sole right to practise euthanasia, society cannot at the same time doubt physicians' conscientiousness. Remarkably, this line of reasoning is widely accepted. Despite decades of sharp criticism of the power of the medical profession, Dutch physicians seem to have gained the unconditional trust of society in matters of life and death.

The core of the new law is the retrospective review procedure. In early

1999, five regional committees had already been established, each consisting of a lawyer (serving as chair), an ethicist and a physician. Each committee judges retrospectively whether the euthanizing physician acted in compliance with the established procedure. Since the new law took effect in April 2002, the public prosecutor can no longer prosecute a euthanasia case if the committee finds that the physician involved has abided by all the requirements of due care. There is also a proposal on the table that covers termination of life without the request of the patient. A national review committee is to be established for such cases, but this proposal has yet to be put into practice. The expectation is that these measures, by diminishing the judicial character of the present procedure, will improve the willingness of physicians to report cases of euthanasia. But the effects of this new review mechanism will only become visible in years to come. Will each committee simply check whether the procedures are satisfied or will it thoroughly investigate each case on the basis of medical, ethical and judicial standards? In the first scenario, the willingness to report cases will certainly increase, but this is far less likely in the second scenario. If the focus is primarily on increasing reporting behaviour, there is a risk of the review of euthanasia becoming a mere bureaucratic routine.

But even if the committees assess each case thoroughly, there remains the problem of the review being retrospective only. It is unclear whether and how this review can curb the practice of euthanasia by preventing the need for euthanasia in the first place. In order to prevent euthanasia, prospective consultation with physicians who are planning to commit euthanasia would have to receive more attention. If palliative care is truly to advance in the Netherlands, professional and institutionalized consultation services will have to be established that precede the decisions of the physicians involved to provide, or not to provide, euthanasia. Creating optimal quality of care for the dying requires easily accessible, prospective palliative care consultation, rather than retrospective case review after the patient has died. Optimal use of expertise in palliative care can make treatment alternatives more visible and in all likelihood decrease the number of euthanasia cases.[87]

Public debate and the politics of compromise

Euthanasia is now a major topic of medical-ethical and legal debate in many countries. The debate in the Netherlands is unusual not only because it started earlier than in other countries, but also because it is a rather open and public debate in which all parties in society participate. The legal context has been a major factor in promoting public debate because no physician committing euthanasia or even ending the life of a patient without the latter's request has ever been sent to prison. Following the 1973 verdict of the District Court of Leeuwarden, public debate on euthanasia in the Netherlands intensified.[88] Concerns about death and dying, and euthanasia in particular, became a media topic. In the second half of 1970 and early 1971, end-of-life issues were being covered and discussed in television documentaries. These programmes fostered a change of mentality and advocated that termination of life in some circumstances should be possible and even desirable.

However, in those early days there was also strong opposition. For example, a 1973 editorial in the *Nederlands Tijdschrift voor Geneeskunde* (Dutch Medical Journal) noted that among the elderly a feeling of uncertainty was growing, discouraging people to visit the physician, fearing that (s)he might terminate their lives.[89] In subsequent 'Letters to the Editor', four replying physicians agreed with the author that euthanasia should be rejected, three disagreed, and one was neutral.

An important watershed was the 1984 publication by the Royal Dutch Medical Association of guidelines for the use of euthanasia in medical practice. In this official position paper, the board of the Medical Association neither advocated nor opposed euthanasia; it merely summarized the conditions for euthanasia as they had been partly defined by the courts. However, by (re)producing the guidelines, the Medical Association de facto accepted the practice of euthanasia; the focus now was on how to regulate it without too much legal interference. The following year, the board decided to establish a committee to study the issue of termination of life without request. This committee was named, without apparent hesitation, Commissie Aanvaardbaarheid Levensbeëindigend Handelen (Committee on the Acceptability of Life-terminating Conduct). The task of this committee was to study if and under which conditions intentional, active termination of life would be acceptable for patients who were not competent to request euthanasia. Twelve years later, when the report was published, the committee concluded that if life-sustaining medical interventions are no longer warranted (e.g. they were no longer beneficial to the patient), active termination of life can be part of the final medical means to assist the patient.[90]

Euthanasia turned into a political issue in 1978.[91] A coalition of members of parliament from six political parties asked the Cabinet to establish a national committee to advise about future policies regarding euthanasia. The ever broader public debate forced the politicians to develop clear views about regulation and policy. In 1982, the Staatcommissie Euthanasie (National Committee on Euthanasia) was established. In its 1985 report, the committee advocated to change the Penal Code. The intentional termination of life should remain punishable but an exception should be codified when the physician ends the life of a patient with unbearable suffering and no prospect for change. One year earlier, the liberal-democratic party (D66) had already submitted a bill to legalize euthanasia in cases where the physician has acted in accordance with the requirements of due care. This bill was then adapted to include the proposals of the National Committee. Although a majority of the political parties seemed to support the bill, it was never passed because the Christian Democratic Party (CDA) opposed. In 1987, however, the government submitted a different proposal to parliament. The proposal stipulated that euthanasia would remain a criminal act and that no exceptions be made. Liability to punishment would be waived only if a euthanizing physician successfully invoked a so-called 'conflict of duties' or *force majeure*, and if certain requirements of due care had been met. The proposal suggested to include these requirements in the Medical Practice Act. However, before a parliamentary discussion could start, the coalition government collapsed.

Euthanasia figured prominently as a political issue in the new elections. The subsequent government, a coalition of the CDA and the PvdA, the socialist Labour Party, decided to initiate a large survey among medical practitioners about the practice of end-of-life decision making. In 1990, a new committee was established (named after its chair, professor of criminal law Remmelink) to supervise this project. In September 1991, the results of the survey were published (for details, see Chapter 3). In November that year, the government submitted a new bill. The Penal Code would not be changed; euthanasia would remain a crime. However, the bill included a new notification procedure for euthanasia cases, developed in cooperation with the Royal Dutch Medical Association.

Although euthanasia would formally remain a crime, this procedure was a first step towards decriminalizing the practice of euthanasia. Previously, the euthanizing physician had only two choices. He could falsify the death certificate by submitting 'death by natural causes', or indicate 'death by non-natural causes', thereby invoking legal proceedings. By changing the Burial Act, the physician would now be able to submit a written report to the medical examiner who would inform the public prosecutor. The latter could then assess whether all requirements of due care were met and, if so, issue a certificate allowing burial or cremation without further investigation. In 1993 this bill was accepted by both houses of parliament. The new law came into force on 1 June 1994. It made the Netherlands the first country to pass explicit legislation on the topic of termination of life.

The new law tried to prevent euthanasia from being viewed as normal medical practice (and hence retained the legal prohibition on any and all terminations of life at the request of the victim), yet facilitate the possibilities for legal audit by increasing the number of reported cases so that the practice could be properly assessed. However, the evaluation of the notification procedure in 1996 did not show any progress. The disappointing result was attributed to the hybrid mixture of penalization and mandatory notification.[92] But by now, a significant change had occurred on the political landscape. After the 1994 elections, the CDA disappeared from government. For the first time since World War II, the Netherlands was governed by a coalition without the Christian Democrats. A new coalition government was formed by the D66, PvdA and the VVD (a conservative-liberal party in the classic sense of that term), parties that had all supported the 1984 D66-draft proposal to legalize euthanasia. The various arguments in favour of legalizing euthanasia were again emphasized. Euthanasia is morally acceptable to a majority of the population, including a majority of medical professionals. Medical acts of terminating life are therefore unjustly criminalized. It was also argued that the criminal law is not effective in accomplishing the purported aims of reporting and auditing. Whereas legal security will not foster the tendency to report, legalizing euthanasia will provide patients as well as physicians with a feeling of protection.[93]

The first thing the new government did was to introduce yet another step to distance the notification procedure from legal control. It established five regional committees to review all reported euthanasia cases. But after gaining another electoral majority and returning to power, this govenment proposed new legislation to legalize euthanasia by physicians altogether. That bill was accepted in 2000 by the Lower House and in 2001 by the Upper House of parliament. It took effect on 1 April 2002.

This overview of the public and political debate demonstrates two features that are often considered characteristic of the Netherlands. First is the quality of public debate. In general, debate on ethical issues is intense and lively in the Netherlands. But the implicit assumption in most debates is that publicity has only advantages. Particularly in regard to euthanasia it is frequently argued that this issue should be debated openly. Physicians performing euthanasia have to come out of the closet. The Dutch have criticized other countries for their hidden euthanasia practice. The basic assumption of public debate is that openness is better than secrecy. It is supposed to be the best remedy against the danger of a slippery slope. This open and liberal climate is also considered an advantage for the practice of health care. As moral theologian Veldhuis has argued: 'People may feel free to discuss their worries about the end of life with their doctors and reach some agreement about the possibility of euthanasia. Just talking about it and expressing their opinions and wishes may already lessen their fears of extreme suffering before dying.'[94] However, Veldhuis has also expressed concern that openness and publicity may increase the number of requests for euthanasia.

The second characteristic is the politics of compromise. The Dutch political system is different from that in two-party systems such as the USA because the citizens elect the members of the Lower House whereas government is formed by the parties winning the elections without any direct involvement from the citizenry. There is always a need for various political parties to make coalitions. We have outlined that legalization of euthanasia only became possible when the electoral outcome in the 1990s forced the exclusion of the Christian Democratic party from government for the first time since World War II. Legal acceptance of euthanasia became a symbolic achievement for the non-Christian parties in the Dutch government of the 1990s.

Of specific significance is the often discussed concept of 'tolerance'. In order to understand the significance of this notion in Dutch politics, we have to step back into history. Because the Dutch Republic in the seventeenth century arose from a coalition of merchants and Calvinist ministers, a curious policy approach emerged, combining the aims of peaceful existence and freedom through policies of tolerance, exemptions and compromises, with the aim of normative regulation of human behaviour through assertion of strict moral standards.[95] This fostered an attitude of pragmatic tolerance. Even if certain kinds of conduct are defined as crimes in the Penal Code, they may end up being regulated officially and tolerated in order to maintain public order. The Penal Code even contains several articles specifying conditions under which a person found guilty of a crime is nevertheless not liable to punishment (see Chapter 4 for a discussion of these articles and their relevance to the euthanasia debate).

This concept of tolerance appears to determine Dutch policies about prostitution, illegal drugs and homosexuality, as well as euthanasia. The moral judgement (that the practice is immoral) is merged with pragmatic considerations (i.e. it cannot be repressed), leading to policies tolerating immoral practices in order to prevent excesses and to control as much as possible existing activities. In recent years, however, there has been a shift towards pluralism. The initial moral judgement is no longer made. Procedure is all that is left. This shift is most evident in the way in which the practice of euthanasia has been dealt with. In the 1980s physicians who committed euthanasia had to prove that they were caught in a conflict of duties. They were let off the hook only if they could convince the court – and yes, the burden of proof was on the physician – that they had been caught in a conflict between the legal prohibition against homicide and the medical obligation to relieve suffering. They had to show that they had been acutely aware of the problematic nature of their conduct by abiding by a series of procedural requirements of due care. But in the 1990s these requirements of due care replaced the conflict of duties: Whenever a physician had abided by the requirements of due care, it was simply assumed that (s)he had also been caught in a conflict of duties and the prosecutor would not even take on the case any more.[96] The non-legal evaluative committees that were established in the late 1990s were no longer expected to assess whether the physician had been caught in a conflict of duties as defined by the criminal code. They only needed to assess whether the physician had abided by the requirements of due care and the prosecutor would simply dismiss the case. Finally, as of 2002, such an assessment by the evaluative committee implies that the physician did not even violate criminal code. The moral judgement that homicide, even at the victim's own request, is immoral has disappeared from view (provided it is a physician who ends the patient's life).

'Human life may be ended by the physician. In two ways. By discontinuing medical treatment, and by performing a medical act. In the first case, the physician is passive ... In the second case, the physician is active. He kills the patient.' We started our historical overview with this quote from Van den Berg.[97] Thirty-three years later, Van den Berg's wishful thinking has become reality. A Dutch physician is indeed allowed to end life in two ways, not only by acquiescing in the patient's impending and inevitable natural death. The physician may also end the patient's life by administering a lethal dose of drugs. In this chapter we have outlined how Van den Berg's outcry against the power of the medical profession paradoxically resulted in a dramatic increase in medical power, the power over life *and death*. We sketched how this could happen historically. But the question remains whether or not this new power of physicians is to be applauded or rejected, whether the ethical arguments in favour of this expansion of power are decisive or rather those against. This is the principal question in the remainder of this book.

3 | The medical practice of euthanasia

Introduction

In Chapter 2 we have seen that euthanasia is generally defined in the Netherlands as 'the intentional termination of the life of a person by someone other than that person at the latter's request'. The definition does not mention either doctors or patients. Granted, many persons who die through euthanasia are patients. They are severely ill or in chronic pain – the domain of physicians. But in the case of euthanasia, the illness is not halted, the patient's life is. Moreover, not all persons dying through euthanasia are 'patients' in the medical sense of that term. As we will see in this chapter, some are simply old and tired of living. Others are unwilling to cope with tragedies. Still others want euthanasia preventively, that is, before cancer or Alzheimer's disease strikes. Hence, for all medical purposes, these persons are still healthy and not in need of medical treatment. Indeed, the Dutch government has repeatedly insisted that euthanasia and assistance in suicide are *not* medical interventions proper, a position espoused once again in its 2002 explanatory brochure about the new euthanasia law.

Yet euthanasia and assistance in suicide have always been the prerogative of physicians in the Netherlands. Whenever lay persons end the life of a beloved family member stricken by terminal illness and begging to be killed, the courts typically have turned against them. Most Dutch citizens believe that euthanasia is justified if and only if it is practised by a physician. The Royal Dutch Medical Association and most Dutch physicians likewise claim the practice as their own. The 2001 law legalizing euthanasia specifically grants this right to physicians and only to them.

At the close of this chapter, we will raise the question as to *why* euthanasia has been medicalized, *why* assistance in suicide has become the prerogative of physicians – a development that is not peculiar to the Netherlands as the English acronym PAS or physician assistance in suicide underscores. But first we will describe and analyse the medical practice of euthanasia and PAS. In the past 25 years, many empirical studies have been undertaken,[98] the results of which are the basis of our analysis. We focus on five themes:

- the incidence of euthanasia and PAS
- the practitioners
- the relationship between patient and practitioner
- the decision-making process
- the retrospective evaluation of the practice by the authorities.

General description of Dutch euthanasia cases

The largest majority of patients who undergo euthanasia or PAS are cancer patients (77 per cent in 2001). Note that cancer was the cause of death for only about a quarter of all Dutch patients in 2001. One out of every 13 cancer patients died as a result of euthanasia/PAS. This is almost ten times more often than all other diseases combined (including such dreaded diseases as chronic obstructive pulmonary disease, AIDS or multiple sclerosis).[99] Although cancer often leads to severe pain, pain was among the reasons to request euthanasia in only 29 per cent of the cases, down from 32 per cent in 1995 and 46 per cent in 1990. The surveyed physicians indicated that preventing pain was among the reasons in 15 per cent of the cases (up from 10 per cent in 1995). In 2001, meaningless suffering (64 per cent), loss of dignity (44 per cent), preventing more severe suffering (36 per cent) and preventing loss of dignity (35 per cent) were much more common reasons.

The performance of euthanasia may occur six months after the patient first asked for it, but it could also take less than a week.[100] In a few cases, the time between request and performance was less than 24 hours.[101] In 1995, roughly half of the patients died within ten minutes of the drugs being administered and most others within one day. The large majority of euthanized patients lose less than one month of life (in 2001 41 per cent lost 1 to 4 weeks and 36 per cent less than a week). Patients who die through PAS tend to be healthier and hence lose more time of life (in 2001, 40 per cent lost more than a month). In a large majority of cases, the patient dies at home (approx. 83 per cent)[102] and it is the patient's family practitioner who ends life (66 per cent of euthanasia cases and 87 per cent of PAS cases in 2001).[103]

Although written euthanasia declarations are becoming ever more popular (43 per cent of all cases in 1990; 70 per cent in 1995; 93 per cent in 2001),[104] little is known about their nature. Euthanasia declarations written long in advance of the need for euthanasia are probably rare. In many instances, patients only complete a written euthanasia declaration when they ask for euthanasia and the physician in turn asks them to write one. They then tend to use the preprinted form prepared by the Dutch Society for Voluntary Euthanasia or a similar standardized form. These forms may tell us more about the physician's keenness to meet the formal requirements of due care than the voluntariness and consideredness of the patient's request. Indeed, the regional review committees charged with the evaluation of euthanasia generally do not assign much weight to them, particularly when a standardized, preprinted form was used.

Whereas euthanasia declarations written by patients are not required by law, the physician is obligated to keep a detailed log. A large majority (85 per cent in 1995) keeps such a log. Consultation with another physician is likewise required and this practice has dramatically increased (from 7 per cent in 1990 to 64 per cent in 1995).[105] Finally, physicians are required to report PAS and euthanasia. By 2001, still only half of all physicians reported to the coroner in spite of a liberal policy of tolerance.

Now that the practice of euthanasia has been described in general terms, we can look at a number of key issues in greater detail. We start with a review of the incidence of euthanasia and PAS.

Incidence of medically procured death (MPD)

Fact or guess?

As explained in the first chapter, there is no term in either the Dutch or the English languages to capture assistance in suicide, euthanasia and all other forms of mercy killing. For ease of reading, we introduce the abbreviation MPD or 'medically procured death' to capture all cases in which the physician strives to hasten the patient's death and directs his/her actions towards that goal. Estimates of MPD have always been remarkably diverse. In 1989, Fenigsen reported estimates ranging from 5000 to 20,000 cases annually. The latter number would equal one in every six or seven patients dying in the Netherlands. Two years later, Van der Maas and colleagues concluded that there were only 2300 euthanasia cases and another 400 cases of assisted suicide. Fenigsen had also claimed many patients were killed without having so requested. His claim was vehemently denied in several Letters to the Editor of the *Hastings Center Report* (1989). Yet two years later, Van der Maas concluded there were indeed about 1000 such cases annually.

Even though much more is known about the practice of euthanasia in the

Netherlands than any other country of the world, any attempt to provide a comprehensive and accurate description of the actual practice of euthanasia and PAS in the Netherlands is bound to fail. One obvious factor contributing to the problem is the illegality of euthanasia and PAS. These practices were illegal in the Netherlands until 2002, and continue to be illegal if practised by anybody other than a physician. Physicians who end the lives of their patients without the latter requesting euthanasia are not immune from prosecution either. It is difficult to survey illegal behaviour accurately, even more so since nobody is obligated to assist in his own prosecution and conviction. MPD is no exception.

But the illegality of these practices is not the only confounding factor. Although illegal, since the mid-1990s, Dutch physicians who practised euthanasia or PAS according to the official governmental guidelines and reported their actions to the authorities were no longer prosecuted. Even those who violated the guidelines had little to fear. Not a single physician has ever been imprisoned for committing euthanasia or assisting in suicide. Physicians found guilty of terminating their patients' lives without a patient request (which legally constitutes murder) were given probationary sentences only (see Chapter 4). Yet despite this policy of legal tolerance towards physicians, the number of reported euthanasia/PAS cases (1466 in 1995; 2054 in 2001) is much lower than the estimated incidence of euthanasia/PAS (3600 in 1995; 3800 in 2001). There could be two causes for this difference. Either many euthanizing physicians – i.e. more than half of them – do not report; or the scientific studies of the practice of euthanasia are flawed, overestimating the incidence of euthanasia. Whatever the cause, the dramatic discrepancy shows that legal tolerance does not necessarily yield empirical clarity.

One of the first to undertake a scientific survey was Van Wijmen and his health law team at the University of Maastricht. He surveyed Dutch physicians about their involvement in euthanasia and PAS in 1983 and 1984. The responses from the 338 family practitioners and specialists who among them had almost 300 cases in each of these two years, would suggest a national incidence of euthanasia/PAS of more than 12,000 cases. A few years later, Van der Wal surveyed the involvement of family practitioners in euthanasia and PAS between 1996 and 1999. He found only about 2000 per year. Van der Wal rejected Van Wijmen's data as unreliable.[106] But on closer inspection, the divergence may have simply been caused by a different definition of euthanasia.

Van Wijmen defined euthanasia as 'intervening or foregoing (of treatment) with the intent to shorten life by a person other than the patient at the latter's request'. He then asked physicians *how* they practised euthanasia and allowed for a variety of answers, such as a lethal injection, increasing the doses of pain medications with the intent to shorten life, forgoing treatment that is not yet futile, and the intentional failure to treat potentially lethal complications. Unlike Van Wijmen, Van der Wal did not include forgoing treatment with the intent to hasten death in his definition of euthanasia. He also excluded specifically the act of increasing pain medications when an additional effect is the shortening of life (the word intent is not mentioned). When Van der Wal enquired about the means to practise euthanasia, he simply assumed this would be done by administering lethal drugs and so he only asked about the kinds and dosages used.

In their large survey study during 1990–91 commissioned by the Dutch government, Van der Maas and colleagues followed Van der Wal and defined euthanasia as intentionally ending the life of another person at the latter's request. Based on this definition, they estimated that 2300 cases or 1.8 per cent of all deaths annually were the result of euthanasia. The research team next asked the surveyed physicians how often they had given very high doses of painkillers knowing the drugs would most likely shorten the patient's life. A large majority of Dutch physicians (80 per cent) had done so at least once, and more than half (58 per cent) had done so in the previous year. In and of itself, these data are not alarming. If patients are in severe pain, physicians are obligated to administer painkillers in spite of those drugs having severe side effects. But the researchers next asked those physicians *why* they had administered the painkillers. Two-thirds of them had done so solely to relieve pain, accepting the life-shortening effect of the drugs as an inevitable side effect. The remaining one-third had done so either to relieve pain *and* shorten the patient's life (30 per cent) or with the sole and express purpose of shortening life (6 per cent).

Van der Maas and colleagues have argued that the last category 'strongly resembles' the practice of euthanasia.[107] We would contend that administering drugs with the sole purpose of shortening the patient's life *is* euthanasia as defined by the researchers, pushing the estimated 1990 incidence of euthanasia up from 2300 to more than 5200. If more than half of euthanizing physicians do not label their own interventions as euthanasia, it becomes very difficult to accurately and comprehensively research and describe the actual practice of euthanasia, let alone regulate the practice.

Bearing in mind these and other confounding factors, in this chapter we will nevertheless attempt to describe the medical practice of MPD in the Netherlands. As mentioned, our statistics are all based on empirical studies undertaken by other scholars. Reinterpreting their numbers in the absence of the original research data is risky.[108] Even though we generally have not rounded our numbers, they are all rough estimates at best.

Empirical studies about the incidence of MPD in the Netherlands

In order to attain more reliable data about the practice of euthanasia and PAS, in 1990 the Dutch government appointed a Committee on the Study of Medical Practice Concerning Euthanasia, also called the Remmelink Committee, named after its president, a prosecutor general for the Supreme Court and professor emeritus of criminal law. The Remmelink Committee faced a daunting task because very little was known about the actual practice of euthanasia when it was established in 1990. As mentioned, in the late 1980s Van Wijmen had analysed 342 questionnaires returned by both family practitioners and specialists about their engagement in MPD in 1983 and 1984. Van Wijmen published his findings in 1989, but only in an internal departmental report. A year later, Van der Wal and colleagues surveyed Dutch family practitioners about their experiences with euthanasia and PAS between 1986 and 1989, but the first results would only come available in 1991.

The Remmelink Committee therefore turned to Professor van der Maas and his colleagues from the Erasmus University of Rotterdam to undertake a large-scale empirical study. The researchers undertook a triple study. First, the team interviewed a sample of 400 physicians about their involvement in euthanasia. Second, it asked the same pool of physicians to complete a short questionnaire for each of their patients who would die in the subsequent six months (the prospective study). Third, the team analysed a representative sample of 8500 death certificates completed in the preceding six months. In those cases where there might have been a medical intervention impacting the time of death, the aforementioned questionnaire was mailed to the attending physician (the retrospective mortality study).

The Remmelink Committee was charged by the government not only to examine the practice of euthanasia, defined as 'any action that intentionally ends the life of someone else, at the request of that person', but also to include all medical decisions in which the physician's purpose is to hasten the patient's death or in which the physician takes into account the probability of hastening the patient's death. This charge is broader in two ways.

First, the committee's expanded charge includes all *decisions* to hasten the patient's death, regardless of whether those decisions are followed by interventions. This also allowed the researchers to study instances of withholding and withdrawing life-sustaining treatment, even if these are not interventions proper but cases of not or no longer intervening.

Second, the report covers not only euthanasia/PAS but also efforts that are more properly characterized as palliative care, such as the provision of adequate pain medications in which the possibility of a hastened death is known but not intended. However, in this chapter we will discuss only the committee's findings that bear on the practice of euthanasia/PAS and related efforts to shorten or end a patient's life purposively (lumped together as MPD).

Incidence of euthanasia and PAS

As pointed out earlier, one of the most remarkable findings of this study by Van der Maas and colleagues (published in 1991) was the low incidence of euthanasia and the even lower incidence of PAS – low, that is, when compared to the estimates that had been circulating in the mass media. Instead of 20,000 cases, there appeared to be only 2300 cases of euthanasia annually and a mere 400 cases of PAS. These numbers coincided with the empirical study by Van der Wal and colleagues.[109] When compared to the 1990 annual mortality (128,824), the number of 2300 euthanasia cases equals 1.8 per cent, and the 400 PAS cases a mere 0.3 per cent. In other words, only 2 out of every 100 patients died as a result of euthanasia or PAS in 1990. However, the numbers change when viewed from the perspective of the physician rather than that of the patient. About one-third of Dutch people die a sudden death due to trauma, cardiac arrest or similar such unexpected or uncontrollable event. Another one-third die under the care of a physician but the issue of delaying or hastening death never surfaces. That leaves some 48,700 cases in which physicians make treatment decisions that impact the patient's time of death. If we compare the 2700 cases of euthanasia/PAS to this number, we find that 1 out of every 18 times physicians decided how to deal with the approaching death of their patients, they decided to hasten death.

The Remmelink Committee concluded that this is still a very low incidence, even more so when one realizes that in 1990 Dutch physicians were confronted with tentative requests for euthanasia some 25,000 times, and with urgent requests 9000 times. Clearly, physicians refuse to hasten death in the large majority of cases. However, elsewhere in the committee's report other forms of intentional hastening of death are listed that change this picture.

Euthanasia under the guise of pain treatment

As mentioned, the committee had decided to examine not only cases of euthanasia and PAS, but also the administration of palliative drugs that can hasten the patient's death. Van der Maas's research team found that in 1990 one out of every three times physicians treated a dying patient, they administered high doses of painkillers in order to relieve the patient's suffering while accepting the potential side effect of a reduced lifespan. But the researchers also uncovered 4500 instances in which painkillers were administered not to relieve the pain but explicitly to hasten the patient's death or among others to hasten death. Here, the reduction of life was no longer an unavoidable and unintended side effect. For these physicians, hastening the death of their patients was an express goal. Indeed, the drugs caused a reduction in patients' lifespans that on average was equal to that reported for the 2300 euthanasia cases.

Did these patients ask for those drugs or at least consent to their administration? The report does not yield an unequivocal answer, but there is evidence that approximately one-third explicitly asked for the painkillers and another one-third was involved in the decision making. Although euthanasia requires an *explicit* request from the patient, we give the physicians involved the benefit of the doubt and label these cases as euthanasia (rather than as cases of nonvoluntary termination of life or – in legal terms – murder). If we next add these cases of 'euthanasia under the guise of pain treatment' to the acknowledged cases of euthanasia and PAS, in 1990 there appear to have been nearly 5600 cases in which physicians granted their patients' wishes to hasten their death by providing or administering lethal doses of drugs or painkillers.

Nonvoluntary termination of life

More troublesome are the cases in which physicians tried to shorten their patients' lives with high doses of painkillers even though the patients themselves had never asked for this and had never been involved in the decision making. The researchers point out that in the large majority of these cases, the patients were incompetent and hence unable to take part in the decision making. Instead, family members were generally consulted. However, euthanasia requires an explicit request from the actual patient. Family members cannot consent to euthanasia on behalf of an incompetent patient. We must therefore label these cases – approximately 1600 in 1990 – as 'nonvoluntary' hastening of the patient's death (not to be confused with 'involuntary' MPD in which the patient's death is hastened *against* the patient's stated wishes).

In the aforementioned 1600 instances, the drugs were administered both to relieve pain and to hasten death. But the researchers also discovered 1000 cases in which drugs were administered solely to end the patient's life without any request from the patient. In some 600 of these 1000 cases, patients had previously expressed the wish to be killed (if, for example, the pain would ever become unbearable or their situation undignified), or they had at some point been involved in the decision making. These cases could therefore be added to the euthanasia tally, increasing that number to roughly 6200. But that leaves 400 cases of nonvoluntary termination of life in which the patient never expressed a wish to be killed and never was asked about this option either.

Some commentators have pointed out that in many of these 400 instances, physicians used morphine and chemically related drugs, which is not a very effective drug if the goal is to end life. Indeed, it is quite difficult to end the life of a patient who has been taking morphine for quite some time by merely increasing the dose. The question hence arises whether these physicians can really be said to have ended their patients' lives.[110] This would certainly be a point of concern for any prosecutor who must prove that the accused has indeed done what he is charged with. In 2001, a prosecutor charged a family physician with providing an 81-year-old patient with 9 grams of pentobarbital. This lethal dose had been requested by the patient for the specific purpose of committing suicide. However, when the deceased was found and an autopsy was performed, too little pentobarbital could be discovered in his blood to prove that the drug had even contributed to the patient's death. On 24 October 2001, the District Court in Assen acquitted the physician for lack of evidence. Courts have to prove that suspects did do what they have been charged with. But the physicians in the 1990 study by Van der Maas admitted that they had increased the morphine and other painkillers in order to hasten death; they certainly intended to hasten death and they themselves believed they were doing so effectively (20 per cent stated death occurred within an hour, another 50 per cent within a day). Even if this could never be proven legally, from an ethical perspective these physicians were engaged in MPD.

Non-treatment decisions

In all of the cases discussed so far, the physician always undertook some action, from prescribing drugs to assisting the patient in her suicide, to overmedicating the patient with painkillers in order to hasten death. The Remmelink Committee also investigated cases in which life-sustaining treatment was withheld or withdrawn. The researchers distinguished three subcategories.

The first subcategory consists of some 10,000 cases in which life-sustaining treatment was withheld or withdrawn because the treatment was unlikely to be effective. In other words, the treatment is not or no longer medically indicated. As the researchers point out, physicians routinely decide to discontinue or forgo treatment when and because it is not or no longer indicated. Although they know that the patient is likely to die subsequently, this is not the physician's intent. It is an inevitable consequence of the incurable disease.

Second, there are cases in which a competent patient refuses life-sustaining treatment. The report shows that almost 71 per cent of physicians interviewed in 1990 had been faced with such a refusal at some point in their medical career. Patients may have many different reasons to do so. They may feel that the side effects render the treatment too burdensome. The treatment proposed may be at odds with their religious beliefs. And some patients may refuse in order to hasten their own death. According to the 1991 report, there may have been as many as 5800 patients in 1990 who refused treatment solely or among others to hasten their own death.[111] The report is not fully clear about the intention of the physicians who granted these patient refusals. The researchers point out that the attending physicians who granted those refusals may themselves not have wanted to hasten death. They may or may not have agreed with the patient's plan to hasten death. We know that approximately two-thirds of patients who refuse life-sustaining treatment do so in order to hasten their own death. We also know that approximately two-thirds of physicians who grant patients' refusals of life-sustaining treatment do so in order to hasten their patients' death. But we do not know for sure whether the former two-thirds coincides with the latter two-thirds.

Legally, the physician's intent is irrelevant because physicians have no choice but to honour a competent patient's refusal of medical treatment, including life-sustaining treatment. But ethically this is an important finding. One could argue that in addition to the cases of *active* euthanasia/PAS in which the physician, at the request of the patient, *actively does* something to hasten the patient's death, there are also cases of *passive* euthanasia/PAS in which the physician, at the request of the patient, does *not* provide treatment in an attempt to hasten the patient's death. A conservative estimate (based on the retrospective study) would indicate that in 1990 there were some 2450 cases of passive euthanasia.

Once again, these cases are legally irrelevant because they would have to be classified as cases in which a competent patient withheld consent for treatment. But that legal line of reasoning does not apply to the third subcategory of patients who died after life-sustaining treatment was withheld or withdrawn. These are cases in which the treatment was medically indicated (i.e. it would have extended life by at least a month), and in which there was no explicit refusal of treatment from the patient, yet it was withheld or withdrawn by the physician anyway. The researchers estimated that this happened some 18,675 times in 1990. In just over half of these cases, the physician was aware that the decision to forgo would shorten the patient's life but did not intend that to happen. There were other reasons to forgo the life-sustaining treatment. However, that leaves some 8350 cases in which hastening death was the very reason to forgo the treatment.

In about 17 per cent of those cases, the physician had discussed with the patient his plan to forgo treatment (and the patient presumably had agreed); in another 13 per cent, the decision had not been discussed with the patient (generally because the patient was incompetent), but the patient had previously expressed a wish for treatment to be forgone in due time. This amounts to an additional 2505 cases of passive euthanasia.

But that still leaves some 5845 cases in which the physician withdrew or withheld life-sustaining treatment in order to hasten death, without any request from or discussion with the patient. Although the patient can legally refuse life-sustaining treatment for any reason, including to hasten death, which refusal must be honoured by the physician, nobody else can legally refuse medical treatment on behalf of the patient in order to hasten death. Suicide, whether by active means or by passively forgoing needed medical treatment, legally is the prerogative of patients. Hence, it does not matter that almost all of these patients were incompetent. All these cases have to be labelled as nonvoluntary termination of life.

Preliminary conclusions

If we table all cases in which physicians' end-of-life care decisions were purposely aimed at shortening the patient's life (see Table 3.1), we find that in 19,000 cases in which physicians cared for dying patients, hastening the patient's death was a goal of treatment planning. Keown performed his own recalculation of the data by Van der Maas et al. and concluded that in 1990 there may have been as many as 26,350 cases of MPD.[112] In short, for every four or five patients who died in 1990 while under the care of a physician, one patient's death has been intentionally hastened by a physician. Note that this is the most conservative estimate. If we compare the number of 19,000 cases to the 48,700 cases in which the possibility of hastening death had to be considered by the attending physician, we find that in 39 per cent of these cases, the physician chose to hasten the patient's death. In short, when Dutch physicians are faced with the option of hastening the patient's death through medical treatment, they choose to do so for three out of every five patients.

In 1995, the 1990 survey was repeated (in somewhat modified form; see Table 3.2). Once again, commentators were quick to point out that the overall incidence of MPD had remained low. Granted, the incidence of euthanasia had increased from 2300 to 3200 cases, reflecting an absolute increase of 0.5 per cent. But then again, the number of PAS cases had remained at 400, and nonvoluntary termination of life had even gone down to 900. But a closer examination of the data again reveals many more forms of MPD that are not officially acknowledged as such. The overall incidence of euthanasia had increased by only 0.2 per cent from 6.8 per cent to 7.0 per cent. The incidence of nonvoluntary termination of life by means of drugs went down by the same 0.2 per cent from 2.2 per cent to 2.0 per cent. However, the number of patients whose lives are intentionally shortened by withholding or withdrawing life-sustaining treatment increased from 5.4 per cent to 9.4 per cent. A similar increase occurred in the number of cases in which physicians decided to forgo life-sustaining treatment in an attempt to shorten life but *without* any request thereto from the patients themselves, rising from 6.4 per cent to 10 per cent. In other words, by 1995 in one in every ten cases in which Dutch physicians cared for dying patients, they

Table 3.1 Medical decisions concerning the end of life (1990 data)

Patient request	Mode	Specification	Number		% of all decisions[1]
Cases of medically procured death (MPD), i.e. cases in which the physician decided to intentionally hasten the patient's death					
Voluntary	Intervening	Physician assisted suicide		400	6.188	6.8

		Active euthanasia
		• Acknowledged as such
		• No explicit request but discussed with
		                              patient
		                              but previous request
		• Under the guise of following explicit
		  pain treatment patient request
		                              no patient request but
		                              discussed
		                              following previous
		                              patient request
			2,300
			
			460
			140
			
			1,339
			
			1,106
			
			443
				5,788	

	Forgoing	Passive euthanasia
		• Following a patient's explicit refusal of
		  treatment
		• After discussion with the patient
		• Following a previous patient wish to forgo
		  treatment
			2,450
			1,420
			
			1,085
				4,955	5.4

Non-voluntary	Intervening	• Mercy killing, acknowledged as such • By means of high doses of painkillers	400 1,612	2,012	2.2
	Forgoing			5,845	6.4
TOTAL				19,000	20.8
Cases in which the probability of hastening death was acknowledged, but the physician's decision was not aimed at hastening the patient's death					
Voluntary	Intervening	Palliative pain treatment • At explicit request of the patient • After discussion with the patient • Following a previous patient wish	2,486 3,723 1,086	7,295	8.0

	Forgoing	• Following a patient's explicit refusal of
		  treatment
		• After discussion with the patient
		• Following a previous patient wish to forgo
		  treatment
			1,375
			1,650
			930
				3,955	4.3

Non-voluntary	Intervening	Palliative pain treatment		10,705	11.7
	Forgoing			7,745	8.5
TOTAL				29,700	32.6
Cases in which the physician's decision about the medical care to be provided did not involve concerns about delaying or hastening the patient's death					
All cases				42,500	46.6
Total of all end-of-life care cases				91,200[1]	100

[1] Total mortality for 1990 was 128,824. However, in approximately 30 per cent, physicians were not involved in the dying process of the patient, e.g. because the patient died after a severe trauma (Van der Maas et al. 1991, p. 155). This leaves approximately 91,200 cases in which physicians made decisions regarding the end of life of their patients.

Table 3.2 Medical decisions concerning the end of life (1995 data)

Patient request	Mode	Specification	Number		% of all decisions[1]
		**Cases of medically procured death (MPD), i.e. cases in which the physician decided to intentionally hasten the patient's death**			
Voluntary	Intervening	Physician assisted suicide		400 · 6,736	7
		Active euthanasia		6,336	
		• Acknowledged as such	3,200		
		• No explicit request but discussed with patient	333		
		but previous request	144		
		• Under the guise of following explicit pain treatment patient request	1,538		
		no patient request but discussed	678		
		following previous patient request	443		
	Forgoing	Passive euthanasia		8,928	9.4
		• Following a patient's explicit refusal of treatment	3,850		
		• After discussion with the patient	3,047		
		• Following a previous patient wish to forgo treatment	2,031		
Non-voluntary	Intervening	• Mercy killing, acknowledged as such	423	1,908	2
		• By means of high doses of painkillers	1,485		
	Forgoing			9,432	10
TOTAL				27,004	28.4
		**Cases in which the probability of hastening death was acknowledged, but the physician's decision was not aimed at hastening the patient's death**			
Voluntary	Intervening	Palliative pain treatment		10,133	10.7
		• At explicit request of the patient	3,124		
		• After discussion with the patient	5,126		
		• Following a previous patient wish	1,883		
	Forgoing	• Following a patient's explicit refusal of treatment	1,350	3,707	3.9
		• After discussion with the patient	1,503		
		• Following a previous patient wish to forgo treatment	854		
Non-voluntary	Intervening	Palliative pain treatment		11,632	12.2
	Forgoing			5,333	5.6
TOTAL				30,805	32.4
		**Cases in which the physician's decision about the medical care to be provided did not involve concerns about delaying or hastening the patient's death**			
All cases				37,191	39.1
Total of all end-of-life care cases				95,000[1]	100

[1] Total mortality for 1995 was 135,675. The 1996 report doesn't indicate in what percentage the researchers estimated physicians not to have played any role. We assume the percentage is approximately the same as in 1990 or 30 per cent. This leaves approximately 95,000 cases in which physicians made decisions regarding patients' end of life.

decided to withhold or withdraw life-sustaining treatment without any request from or involvement by the patients themselves.

In 2003, yet another update of the 1990 study was published by Van der Wal. The published report contains far fewer details about the practice of MPD (and more about the evaluation of the practice and public attitudes about MPD). This hampers a comparison with the 1990 and 1995 data. Overall, the incidence of acknowledged euthanasia (3500) and PAS (300) and various other forms of MPD remained roughly the same between 1995 and 2001. In fact, a small overall decrease in the incidence of MPD is noticeable (down from 28.4 per cent in 1995 to 26.5 per cent in 2001). Conversely, the total number of cases in which the probability of hastening death was acknowledged but the physician's decisions were *not* aimed at hastening the patient's death increased considerably from 32.4 per cent of all end-of-life care cases in 1995 to 36 per cent in 2001 (Table 3.3).

The most noticeable changes between 1995 and 2001 concern the practice of nonvoluntary MPD and the provision of genuine palliative care. The significant rise in cases of nonvoluntary MPD between 1990 (8.6 per cent) and 1995 (12 per cent) had halted by 2001 (11.3 per cent). Whereas in 1995 55 per cent of physicians were willing to end a patient's life without an explicit request from the patient, by 2001 only 29 per cent of physicians were still willing to do so. In 1990, more than a quarter (27 per cent) of all physicians had once ended a patient's life without a patient request. By 2001, only 13 per cent had once done so. This suggests that younger physicians are ever more hesitant to do so. On the other hand, the provision of genuine palliative care that acknowledges the danger of shortening life but never aims at such a reduction, increased as well from 19.7 per cent in 1990 to 22.9 per cent in 1995 and to 25.9 per cent in 2001.

Who practises euthanasia?

The incidence of euthanasia and PAS increased steeply in the 1980s, to 2700 cases in 1990 and more gradually to 3800 cases in 2001. Thus, there may have been some 55,000 cases of euthanasia/PAS in the last two decades of the twentieth century combined. Bearing in mind a gradual increase in the number of Dutch physicians in the same period, on average physicians should have had one case of euthanasia/PAS every three years. However, the literature suggests that the frequency with which Dutch physicians practise euthanasia/PAS differs tremendously. Consider the eight family practitioners who shared their stories in *Asking to Die*.[113] One of these physicians had never committed euthanasia in his 30 years of practice; 6 physicians had practised euthanasia between five and nine times in their 15 to 20 years of practice; one refused to reveal how many times he had practised euthanasia but admitted having been a consultant some 300 to

Table 3.3 Medical decisions concerning the end of life (2001 data)

Patient request	Mode	Specification	Number			% of all decisions[1]
Cases of medically procured death (MPD), i.e. cases in which the physician decided to intentionally hasten the patient's death						
Voluntary	Intervening	Physician assisted suicide		300	5,881	6

		Active euthanasia
		• Acknowledged as such
		• No explicit request but discussed with
		                                      patient
		                                      but previous request
		• Under the guise of pain treatment[2]
			3,500
			255
			98
			1,728
				5,581		

	Forgoing	Passive euthanasia[3]			9,030	9.2
Non-voluntary	Intervening	• Mercy killing, acknowledged as such[2] • By means of high doses of painkillers[3]		627 972	1,644	1.7
	Forgoing				9,400	9.6
TOTAL					25,955	26.5
Cases in which the probability of hastening death was acknowledged, but the physician's decision was not aimed at hastening the patient's death						
Voluntary	Intervening (i.e. palliative pain treatment)[4]				12,000	12.2
	Forgoing[5]				4,060	4.1
Non-voluntary	Intervening (i.e. palliative pain treatment)[4]				13,500	13.7
	Forgoing[5]				5,860	6
TOTAL					35,420	36
Cases in which the physician's decision about the medical care to be provided did not involve concerns about delaying or hastening the patient's death						
All cases					36,825	37.5
Total of all end-of-life care cases					98,200[1]	100

[1] Total mortality for 2001 was 140,377. The 2001 report doesn't indicate in what percentage the researchers estimated physicians not to have played any role. We assume the percentage is approximately the same as in 1990 or 30 per cent. This leaves approximately 98,300 cases in which physicians made decisions regarding patients' end of life.

[2] In 1990, 64 per cent of MPD with pain medications were voluntary; in 1995, 64 per cent. No information is available for 2001. The 2001 report states that no important changes had taken place since 1995 (p. 68). Hence we use the 1995 percentages.

[3] In 1990, 46 per cent for MPD by forgoing cases were voluntary; in 1995, 49 per cent. No information is available for 2001. The 2001 report states that no important changes had taken place since 1995 (p. 68). Hence we use the 1995 percentages.

[4] In 1990, 41 per cent of palliative cases were voluntary; in 1995, 47 per cent. No information is available for 2001. The 2001 report states that no important changes had taken place since 1995 (p. 68). Hence we use the 1995 percentages.

[5] In 1990, 33 per cent for forgoing cases were voluntary; in 1995, 41 per cent. No information is available for 2001. The 2001 report states that no important changes had taken place since 1995 (p. 68). Hence we use the 1995 percentages.

350 times. Dr van Oijen, who figured in the internationally televised documentary about one of his own cases, averaged three cases per year by 1994.[114] In the same year, the Central Medical Disciplinary Court of Appeals dealt with a physician who worked for the Dutch Society for Voluntary Euthanasia (NVVE). In less than five months, she had ended the life of a demented patient, euthanized a second patient, and assisted in the suicide of a third.[115] We find a similar variance for specialists who practise in hospitals. Whereas one university medical centre hospital had had a few

dozen cases of euthanasia by 1997,[116] another had had 2000 to 3000 cases of euthanasia in the same period.[117]

More striking perhaps is that by 2001, 43 per cent of all Dutch physicians had still *never* been involved in euthanasia.[118] Apparently, the same contingent of Dutch physicians has been responsible for all of the euthanasia throughout the years, each averaging two cases every three years. The earliest indicators that this hypothesis is correct are found in the 1989 study by Van Wijmen. He discovered that 62.1 per cent of the surveyed physicians had not a single case of euthanasia in 1983 and again, 63 per cent had no case in 1984. Conversely, in 1983, 10 per cent of the physicians were responsible for half of all the euthanasia cases and half the PAS cases, and again in 1984. One physician reported ten euthanasia cases in 1983 and the same happened in 1984.

Van der Wal's research over the period 1986 to 1989 shows the same phenomenon.[119] In that four-year period, 6296 Dutch family practitioners were jointly responsible for 7996 cases of euthanasia and PAS. This would suggest one case in every three to four years per family practitioner. But the reality is quite different. More than half of the physicians (53 per cent) did not have a single case of euthanasia in all four years. That pushes the average per euthanizing physician up to two cases for every three years. But even within this group, there are significant differences: 30 per cent of the euthanizing physicians was responsible for 35 per cent of the cases; another 12 per cent was responsible for yet another 35 per cent; and the remaining 30 per cent of the cases was performed by only 5 per cent of Dutch family practitioners. The real distribution therefore is as follows:

- 53 per cent had no case of euthanasia/PAS in four years
- 30 per cent had a single case every three years
- 12 per cent had one case per year
- 5 per cent averaged two cases per year.

The trend continues. The 1991 study by Van der Maas shows that about a quarter (24 per cent) of Dutch physicians were responsible for all euthanasia/PAS cases in 1989–90, averaging one case annually for each of them. By 1990, 46 per cent of Dutch physicians had never had a case of euthanasia or PAS. The follow-up study by Van der Wal and Van der Maas (1996) shows that just over one quarter (29 per cent) of Dutch physicians had been responsible for all of the euthanasia/PAS cases in 1994–5 whereas 47 per cent still had not had a single case in the course of their practice. As mentioned, by 2001 43 per cent still had never had a case of euthanasia whereas 30 per cent were responsible for all cases in 2000–01, each averaging slightly more than one case per year. Among hospital-based specialists, the variance is even greater. Their 1900 cases of euthanasia in 1994–5 were performed by only 16 per cent of the specialists or 500 doctors, each averaging two cases per year. In 2000–01, specialists averaged three cases per two years.

What can explain this striking variance among Dutch physicians? One obvious possibility would be the willingness of Dutch physicians to practise euthanasia. But the statistics show that this cannot be the primary cause of the variance. Only 11 per cent of all Dutch physicians refuse to practise euthanasia/PAS (up from 8 per cent in 1990 and 9 per cent in 1995). That leaves 32 per cent who are willing to practise, yet by 2001 have not had a single case in the course of their careers. If we assume that it was but a matter of chance that they did not have a case, the following breakdown arises:

- 11 per cent of Dutch physicians refuse to practise euthanasia
- 67 per cent average at most one case every 18 years
- 17 per cent have one case annually and are responsible for more than half of all cases each year
- 5 per cent average two cases annually and are responsible for a third of all cases of euthanasia each year.

If the variance cannot be explained by the willingness of the physicians, maybe some physicians simply never get asked by their patients to commit euthanasia. There is probably some truth in this hypothesis because 27 per cent of Dutch family practitioners did not have a single request for PAS/euthanasia between 1986 and 1989.[120] But then again, by 2001, 99 per cent of Dutch family practitioners stated that they had received one or more requests at some point in their career. And 90 per cent of all family practitioners (77 per cent of all physicians combined) had received one or more urgent requests. One family practitioner who by 1995 had never practised euthanasia indicated that he receives about one request per year.[121] But even this number is remarkably low. In 2001, family practitioners received almost 25,000 requests which translates to three to four requests per practitioner per year.[122]

If almost all physicians are asked for euthanasia, some more often than others, why is it that a relatively small contingent of physicians ends up with a large majority of the PAS/euthanasia cases, whereas a large majority almost always refuses to grant those requests? The 1995 data show that the competence of patients who make requests is not decisive either. Most requests for euthanasia were refused in spite of the request being quite explicit (approximately 75 per cent) and the patients being fully able to make decisions about euthanasia (62 per cent). In only 6 per cent of refused requests were patients deemed incompetent due to dementia or mental disability.

Is the difference between those physicians who frequently euthanize patients and those who never do (despite being willing and asked by competent patients) the result of certain physicians treating more seriously ill patients with poorer prognoses? If this would be the case, one would expect the lowest frequency among family practitioners, a higher frequency among specialists working in hospitals, and the highest incidence of euthanasia among nursing clinic physicians who treat mostly elder patients with chronic, irreversible and debilitating conditions that require institutional care. Remarkably, the frequencies are exactly reverse. By 2001, 71 per cent of family practitioners had practised euthanasia, but only 37 per cent of hospital-based specialists and 36 per cent of nursing clinic physicians. In the period 2000–2001, 38 per cent of family practitioners committed euthanasia, but only 16 per cent of hospital-based specialists and 21 per cent of Dutch nursing clinic physicians did.

These numbers suggest that the variance is not the result of differences in the medical condition of the patients either. This conclusion is further supported by the fact that there is a striking variance within each category of physicians. Consider the category of family physicians. It is unlikely that two-thirds of Dutch family practitioners did not care for dying patients in 2001–02. It is certainly impossible that one-third of all willing family practitioners had no potential euthanasia case in two decades when the other two-thirds on average had ten cases in the same period. One nursing clinic physician has explained the low incidence of euthanasia among his colleagues as follows: 'A reason for this is that sometimes when a patient is told that euthanasia is possible, he or she feels at ease and goes on to die naturally.' But this reasoning should apply likewise to the patients of family practitioners and hospital-based specialists. He then goes on to explain that nursing clinic physicians are 'a little more conservative than the general practitioner and we tend to protect our patients more because they are weaker. The general practitioner ascribes enormous responsibility to the patient's own health behaviour. As nursing home physicians, we are much more protective.'[123]

The latter explanation is intriguing because it suggests that one of the main reasons for the variance in the frequency with which Dutch physicians practise euthanasia is their variant understanding of the doctor–patient relationship. Many physicians who are not in principle opposed to euthanasia nevertheless take it to be their obligation to protect patients against their own despair and weakness. Consequently, they are much less likely to grant a request for euthanasia. Conversely, some physicians believe that the patient's request is decisive; if patients ask for euthanasia, their request must be granted.

In Chapter 2, we have seen that family practitioners ever since the 1960s have claimed to relate differently to their patients. Does this difference in understanding of the doctor–patient relationship impact the PAS/euthanasia practice? In 2001–02, family practitioners got roughly 13,000 requests for 'euthanasia in the near future'. Of these requests, 40 per cent were granted. Hospital-based specialists granted 37 per cent of the urgent requests they received and nursing clinic physicians 41 per cent. This would suggest family practitioners, hospital-based specialists and nursing clinic physicians are about equally paternalistic.

The doctor–patient relationship

It is difficult to get a clear sense of the nature of the Dutch doctor–patient relationship in the context of euthanasia because no systematic empirical research has been undertaken in this area. However, a number of physicians engaged in euthanasia have written about their experiences. In *Asking to Die*, Thomasma and co-authors include as many as 12 first-person narratives by euthanizing physicians and two more interviews. Though diverse in many regards, several shared characteristics can be discerned.

First, these physicians take it for granted that it is their obligation as physician to provide euthanasia. Although they insist that the patient has to be absolutely certain that (s)he wants euthanasia, they do not appear to perceive a need to justify their own committing euthanasia. All physicians insist that the practice of euthanasia is always tense, difficult, exhausting; but they are also certain they did the right thing each time. They are 'at peace' with their decisions.[124] As one physician states: 'I never have trouble sleeping or experience remorse; instead I feel satisfied that I have done the best I could to help my patient.'[125] This conviction of righteousness is mirrored by their anger about the need to defend their actions to legal authorities as if they are criminals.[126] The same physician goes on to state that the only case about which he was and continues to be troubled is one in which he did *not* grant the patient's wish. Subsequently, the patient refused to eat or drink and died four days later: 'This is the only case I have regretted – because she really meant it when she asked me to help her die, and she was stronger than I was in carrying it out.'[127] It should be pointed out that this physician's reasons for not granting the patient's wish was his belief that she was depressed. In due time, she might overcome the depression and enjoy her life again even though confined to her bed. After all, she did not have intractable pain. Nevertheless, this physician continues to worry that he abandoned the patient and in fact harmed her by not ending her life.

These quotes lead us to a second characteristic shared by the physicians who wrote about their own involvement in euthanasia. They are all convinced that the patient's autonomy trumps the physician's duty to be beneficent. It is up to the patient to choose in favour of life or in favour of death, and it would be wrong for the physician to block that choice. One physician asked rhetorically: 'Should I have said, "I still have more morphine to comfort you with, you are not suffering enough, and according to the books it's not time to die yet"? To do so would be a violation of the understanding between physician and patient.'[128] In other words, euthanasia becomes an act of beneficence and the refusal to do so a violation of the old medical-ethical maxim *primum non nocere*, first and foremost do not harm. Said one physician: 'Despite the seeming contradiction with the doctor's professional injunction "Do No Harm", it seemed clear to me that euthanasia for this patient would not be doing him harm. I had to conclude that he remains steadfast in wanting to die, the moment will come when I can only love him by killing him.'[129]

As pointed out earlier, one physician believed his patient was the stronger one, whereas he faintheartedly took too much time. Another physician talked about his initially not daring to do it, lacking the strength to help his patient. Yet another expressed his admiration for the way in which some of his patients took charge in an almost heroic manner: 'Pieter, for example, in his professional life was a middle-level administrator for a public utility company. Although a very active and alert man, he never reached notable achievements. When it came time to plan how he wanted to die, he was a giant in my eyes. He attained a stature in death that he never had in life. There have been other example too, where people outgrew their own pettiness and limitations.'[130]

The foregoing quotes not only suggest a leading role for the patients in decision making about euthanasia. Some phrases in these narratives show the physicians involved were drawn too deeply into their patients' misery and suffering, thereby breaching the necessary therapeutical distance. Most physicians who practise euthanasia – though not all – know their patients quite well. They have cared for them many years, attended to them at their homes, and may address one another with first names (rather than Dr X and Mrs B). But there is a fine line between effective communication and empathic communion. One physician recounted how his patient, upon expressing a wish for euthanasia, insisted that they now switch to such more informal communications.[131] Another wrote: 'My patient's plight invades every aspect of my thinking ... As I am drawn closer and closer to really understanding my patient's plight, not in technical terms but in the very way the circumstances affect that individual patient, I feel myself in that patient's place. I can imagine how it is for them, how it feels when living is worse than dying.'[132] Dr Chabot, the psychiatrist who assisted in the suicide, admitted that his decision to assist her in spite of her depression lay in her 'extraordinary personality ... She was such a strong and sensitive person at the same time.'[133]

These quotes from *Asking to Die* suggest that the decision in favour of euthanasia is always the patient's prerogative, maybe at times even too much the patient's prerogative. The physician's role in this process is secondary and limited to providing information, clarifying, counselling, but never deciding paternalistically on behalf of the patient. In contrast, physicians who seldom or never practise euthanasia do not attribute as much weight to patient autonomy. We already quoted the nursing clinic physician who alleged that his colleagues often assume a more paternalistic stance in order to 'protect' the patient against her own weakness. Although we have not been able to determine which medical disciplines harbour more paternalistic physicians, the data from the three empirical studies (from 1990, 1995, 2001) suggest that medical paternalism is much more prevalent than is usually claimed by Dutch proponents of euthanasia.

The physician's role in the decision-making process

The Dutch government (when it legalized euthanasia and PAS in 2001), the Royal Dutch Medical Association and the various Dutch pro-euthanasia associations have always underscored the decisive significance of the patient's request. The request has even become part of the very definition of euthanasia in the Netherlands. But the discussion in the preceding section suggests the role of the physician is actually quite important in the decision-making process, maybe even more important than that of the patient. The anthropological studies of the Dutch euthanasia practice in different Dutch hospitals by The and Pool show that the decision-making process leading up to the actual event is one of negotiation between patient and physician (as well as several other parties such as nurses and family members). A recent book on Dutch euthanasia is aptly titled *Regulating Physician-Negotiated Death*.[134]

Initiation of the euthanasia request

Consider the initial request for euthanasia. When surveyed in 1995, 99 per cent of Dutch physicians engaged in euthanasia claimed the request was fully initiated by the patient.[135] Yet at the same time, 56 per cent of all surveyed physicians also believed that in certain circumstances it is appropriate for a physician to propose euthanasia as an option to the patient (rather than wait for the patient to ask for euthanasia).[136] In 1995, almost 53 per cent of all Dutch physicians had already performed euthanasia or PAS and 35 per cent were willing to do so, leaving only 12 per cent who would never practise euthanasia or PAS themselves. When asked about their willingness to end a patient's life without an explicit request from the patient, 45 per cent indicated a principled unwillingness to do so, leaving still more than half of Dutch physicians willing to do so. More importantly, we already saw that in 1995 there were almost 2000 cases in which patients' lives were ended by physicians by means of drugs *without* a request from the patient and almost 10,000 cases in which life-sustaining treatment was withheld in order to hasten death, again *without* a request from the patient. About one-third of the physicians involved in these cases thought they already knew what the patient wanted. The latter number had almost doubled since 1990 (from 17 per cent to 30 per cent).

By 2001, only 29 per cent of Dutch physicians were still willing to end life without an explicit patient request. The incidence of nonvoluntary MPD had gone down from 12 per cent to 11.3 per cent. But that still means that more than 11,000 patients' lives were ended without any request from the patients involved.

Persistence of the request

If we compare the statistics for requests versus granted cases, another interesting phenomenon becomes visible. In 1994–5, some 14,500 requests for 'euthanasia in due time' were directed to Dutch hospital-based specialists. However, we also know that most of these 14,500 requests did not become persistent. In 1994–5, there were only 6000 requests for 'euthanasia in the near future'. We furthermore know that 16 per cent of all specialists, about 500 of them, were responsible for the roughly 1680 cases of euthanasia requests granted in that same period. Most likely, these specialists did not grant every request they received. If we assume that they granted half of the requests they received (see also p. 79), they must have received 3360 urgent requests or almost seven each. That leaves 2654 urgent requests for the remaining specialists. Since 36 per cent of specialists had never yet had an urgent request (and hence no such request in 1994–5 either), the remaining specialists averaged one request each. The 2000–01 statistics show a similar pattern. The 16 per cent of specialists who practised euthanasia in those two years averaged about six requests each; 41 per cent of specialists received one request, whereas the remaining specialists received no request at all during those two years. That pattern is even more pronounced among family practitioners. In 2000–01, euthanizing physicians received six times as many requests as their non-euthanizing colleagues.

We thus find that euthanizing physicians get more requests than physicians who are willing to practise euthanasia (or at least refer) but do not do so. Euthanizing physicians also end up with far more initial requests becoming persistent. One can easily understand that physicians who actually practise euthanasia are asked to become consultants much more frequently than those who have never practised euthanasia. But it is less clear why physicians who practise euthanasia get asked more often by their patients. And more importantly, why it is that the patients of physicians who practise euthanasia tend to persist more in their request for euthanasia than patients of physicians who do not practise euthanasia, though they are willing to do so. The only logical explanation for this variance is that some physicians strengthen their patients' desire for euthanasia, whereas other physicians manage to guide patients to other alternatives.

Acceptance or refusal of the request

Once the patient's request for MPD has become urgent and persistent, the physician must decide whether or not to grant that request. In 1995 there were far more cases of persistent requests for euthanasia that were *not* executed than executed. About half of these unmet requests simply were not met because the patient died before MPD could be executed. But that still leaves about 3000 instances in which the patients' persistent requests were not granted by their physicians, almost as many instances in which requests were granted (3600 cases).[137] In 2001, about 2500 urgent persistent requests were not granted by the physicians involved (compared to 3800 granted cases).

If we look at the reasons given by the physicians who refused in 1995, we find first of all that about one-third of the patients according to their physicians were not fully competent to make the decision in favour of MPD (because of dementia, mental handicaps, depression or some other psychiatric disturbance). Since both euthanasia and PAS by definition require that the patient is competent, one would have to conclude that these cases simply would not have qualified as euthanasia had the physician granted the request, but as nonvoluntary termination of life cases. That leaves about 2000 cases in which a fully competent patient had expressed a persistent and urgent request for euthanasia, and yet the attending physician refused to grant the request.

In about 10 per cent of these cases, the physician refused because the patient's freedom to choose had been reduced; for example, by the pressure exerted by family members. Again, one would have to argue that had these physicians granted the request for MPD, their actions could not have been labelled as euthanasia, but only as nonvoluntary termination of life. The same is true for the 16 per cent of patients who, according to the attending physician, did not have an adequate insight into the nature of their own illness. Whenever a patient asks for euthanasia without having been properly informed, this request is not well considered. And any patient who, in spite of proper information, still does not understand the nature of his/her illness, is legally incompetent to consent to a medical intervention.

What, then, were the reasons of the physicians who refused to honour the requests for euthanasia by their fully free, informed and competent patients? A very small number of these refusals occurred because the physician had principled objections (4 per cent; down from 19 per cent in 1990). Another small minority (6 per cent) refused because they feared legal consequences – a rather strange reason given that in the five years preceding the 1995 study, only two out of every 1000 physicians engaged in MPD were prosecuted and not a single Dutch physician has ever gone to jail for ending his patient's life. This leaves us with four different reasons given to refuse. In about one-third of all refused cases (or 1000 cases), according to the physicians there were alternative ways of relieving the patient's suffering. This is an important ground for refusing euthanasia because the law has always required that the patient's suffering must be without prospects.

It is only reasonable to assume that in these cases, the patient was not willing to try those alternatives or, unlike the physician, was not satisfied with the results of those interventions. For otherwise the patient would not have persisted in her request for euthanasia/PAS. But if so, why did their physicians not execute the request? In the final resort it is up to the patient to determine whether the alternatives are worth trying. If they are not, they are not reasonable alternatives, thus the Explanatory Note to the new law.[138] The physician can then proceed and legally execute the euthanasia request. Indeed, in 12 per cent of the cases of euthanasia/PAS that *were* granted, there were still effective alternatives according to the physician, but the patient had refused them, insisting on euthanasia instead. We thus find that in 1995, there were about 1430 patients who persisted in their request for euthanasia in spite of effective alternatives being available to relieve their suffering. The question now arises why in one-third of these cases, physicians granted the request and in two-thirds they refused. These refusing physicians were certainly within their right to do so. No physician is ever obligated to grant a patient's request for euthanasia, even more so when there are effective alternative means to relieve the patient's suffering. But the fact remains that a large majority of the physicians involved opted for a paternalistic course of action instead of respecting the autonomous wishes of their fully competent patients.

The second reason given to refuse the patient's request was that the patient's suffering was still bearable. The 1995 study by Van der Wal and colleagues showed that in 35 per cent of all refused cases (about 1000 cases), this was one of the reasons to refuse. Subsequent research by Haverkate and colleagues revealed that the patients' suffering according to their physicians was still bearable in 70 per cent of the refused cases; the suffering was moderately unbearable in 19 per cent and very much unbearable in 11 per cent of the cases. Among granted cases, the statistics were 17 per cent, 25 per cent and 58 per cent respectively.[139] Again, the bearableness of suffering is an important and valid reason to refuse euthanasia because the patient's suffering must be both prospectless and unbearable. But unlike the former, the latter is not an objective medical criterion. On the basis of objective scientific information, the physician can judge whether there is still prospect for improvement through effective medical means to relieve suffering. But only the patient can determine whether her suffering is bearable. This difference has been emphasized throughout the public and legal debates on euthanasia and underlies the persistent use by the courts and the legislature of two separate require-ments: the patient's suffering must be prospectless *and* unbearable. Two possible scenarios thus arise:

1 A competent patient persisted in her request for euthanasia, but admitted that her suffering was still bearable. The physician then responded that it was fully up to her to determine whether the suffering was still bearable, but as long as she insisted it was bearable, he could not grant her request for euthanasia/PAS.

But this is not a very probable scenario. More likely is that:

2 the patient persisted in her request for euthanasia/PAS but the physician concluded that the patient's suffering was still bearable such that her request for euthanasia/PAS was not urgent enough to be granted.

This second scenario must have played itself out about 1000 times in 1995. Given Dutch insistence that the judgement about the (un)bearableness of suffering is the sole prerogative of patients, one can only conclude that many physicians paternalistically overrode their patient's judgement.

The third reason given to refuse euthanasia were objections on the part of the physician involved against euthanasia in this particular case. This rea-son was given by 20 per cent of the refusing physicians, representing some 600 cases in 1995. This third and very vague reason again smacks of medical paternalism.

The fourth and last reason was 'other'. We will not speculate what those 'other' reasons might have been and whether they too are suggestive of medical paternalism. But we do note that there were 'other' reasons to refuse euthanasia in 17 per cent of cases in 1995 (11 per cent in 1990; 14 per cent in 2001). We find it rather troublesome that so many physicians have reasons to refuse euthanasia that the researchers studying them cannot even predict. If so much ambiguity persists about what motivates physicians to grant or refuse euthanasia, it becomes very difficult to guide and regulate the practice of MPD through policy or law – an issue we will return to in the final chapter.

Execution of the request

Although for some patients deciding in favour of MPD may be more dif-ficult than undergoing it later on, from an ethical and legal perspective the execution of MPD is the most crucial moment. As long as doctor and patient only discuss and plan MPD, no illegal act has been committed. It is only when a lethal drug is taken and the patient dies as a result that a homicide occurs. This is the moment of irreversibility. It is also the moment of ultimate responsibility. From an ethical and legal perspective it therefore makes a difference who commits this ultimate act. Is it the patient who takes the lethal drugs himself and thereby takes final responsibility for his own death? Or is it the doctor who injects the lethal drugs, and thereby takes final responsibility? If the physician merely assists in the patient's own suicide, her role is exactly that: assistance. Whenever somebody assists in an act, be it a bad or a good act, she cannot and may not take full credit for the act. The dealer who sold the stolen car that was used as a get-away vehicle in a bank robbery cannot be convicted for the bank robbery itself. The pharmacist who mixed the paints for Michelangelo cannot take credit for the Sistine Chapel. Likewise, the physician who provides a patient with lethal drugs is not equally responsible for the ensuing death as the patient who swallows the drugs. Conversely, if the physician injects the drugs herself, he carries final responsibility even if the patient asked for those drugs. This difference is reflected in Dutch law. Assisting in a suicide is punishable with up to three years of imprisonment; ending another person's life at his request is punishable with up to 12 years (for a more extensive discussion of the difference between euthanasia and PAS, see Chapter 5).

In the Netherlands (and elsewhere as well), patient self-determination and freedom of choice have always been advanced as decisive ethical justifications for MPD. If we grant this, it logically follows that the practice of PAS is ethically preferable to euthanasia. Autonomy implies responsibility. The patient's freedom to choose against life and in favour of death implies that the patient also assumes final responsibility for this gravest of choices. This line of reasoning has led the US state of Oregon to legalize PAS only; euthanasia has remained a crime.

However, the Dutch empirical studies from the 1980s and 1990s as well as the 1998 to 2002 annual reports from the five Regional Review Committees that assess each reported case of MPD consistently show that euthanasia is practised about ten times more often than PAS. Why this remarkable difference? The earliest study by Van Wijmen provides some insight. Physicians are much less willing to practise PAS. They tend to view requests for PAS more often as a sign that the patient is suffering from a mental illness and/or incompetent.[140] Unfortunately, all subsequent studies simply lumped PAS and euthanasia together and treat them as if they are the same.

One possible explanation of the preponderance of euthanasia would be that most patients who ask for MPD are no longer able to commit suicide, even with the assistance of a physician. They can no longer swallow the drugs; or if they can, they might throw up and emit the drugs again. Even though there may be some cases, it seems quite unlikely that this would be true for 90 per cent of the patients. As mentioned, no empirical studies are available that assess this explanation, but one family practitioner wrote that in only 10 per cent of his cases was there a need to intravenously inject the lethal drugs (i.e. commit euthanasia). All other patients were able to take the drugs orally (i.e. commit suicide).[141]

A second possibility would be that most patients ask physicians for euthanasia instead of PAS. Van Wijmen's study confirms this hypothesis. The 337 physicians in his sample together received not quite 100 requests for PAS in 1983 and again in 1984, but more than 360 requests for euthanasia.[142] Likewise, Van der Wal found that between 1986 and 1989 family practitioners received 3.5 times as many requests for euthanasia than PAS.[143] Many patients probably ask for euthanasia instead of PAS precisely because euthanasia shifts the final responsibility from the patient to the physician. Ending one's own life, even if it is burdened by pain and suffering, is a very difficult decision. Patients may feel somewhat relieved when their physician is willing to end their life for them, thereby assuming final responsibility for this act. Arentz recounts how several of his patients became fully conscious of the magnitude of their request for euthanasia only when he volleyed the question back at them, asking the patient to bear the final responsibility by ingesting the lethal drugs.[144]

But Arentz clearly is the exception among Dutch physicians. Most of his colleagues do not insist that patients bear the final responsibility for their autonomous choices. Instead, the large majority of physicians simply assume that responsibility for them, allowing the patient the more comfortable role of passive victim. Even if these physicians do not intend to limit the autonomy of their patients, their paternalistic behaviour de facto curbs it.

Evaluation of the practice of euthanasia

Reporting

The number of cases reported to the combined prosecutors shows an exponential increase over the final two decades of the twentieth century. This increase in reporting can be explained in part by the increase in the actual incidence of euthanasia/PAS, for we have seen that the incidence grew from 2700 cases in 1990 to 3600 in 1995 and 3800 in 2001. However, the reporting data do not show a linear increase. There is a very steep increase in 1991 and 1992, and again in 1996 to 1998. Although it is theoretically possible that in these years the actual incidence of euthanasia/PAS increased dramatically, it is more likely that the incidence of euthanasia increased steadily between 1990 and 1995, but the willingness on the part of physicians to report jumped in 1991 and 1992, then tapered off, and augmented again in 1996 to 1998, tapering off again in the late 1990s. This sudden augmentation in the willingness to report coincides with the publication of the first national euthanasia surveys in 1991 and 1996 respectively.

If we extrapolate the annual increase in the incidence of euthanasia and PAS between 1990 and 1995 to the five years preceding 1990, we find that the willingness to report slowly increased in the 1980s to 18 per cent in 1990. Indeed, Van Wijmen found that only 5 per cent of the physicians in his sample reported between 1983 and 1984.[145] Van der Wal's study from 1992 showed that in the province of North Holland, the reporting incidence among family practitioners grew from 8 per cent in 1986 to 18 per cent in 1989. The reporting incidence next jumped to 39 per cent in 1992, stabilizing in the subsequent years at about 44 per cent in 1995. It then jumped again to 62 per cent, followed by a gradual decrease back to 54 per cent in 2001 (Figure 3.1).

Figure 3.1 Reporting of euthanasia

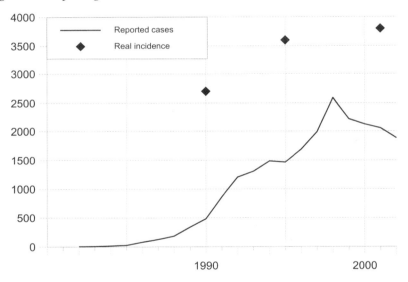

The reasons *not* to report are varied. Many physicians continue to complain that it is too much of a hassle to report: 55 per cent of physicians gave this as a reason not to report in 1995[146] (although this negative view had decreased by about half in 2001).[147] Moreover, among those who did not report, only 11 per cent had taken the trouble to consult with another physician (compared to 94 per cent of those who did report), and only 57 per cent had made written notes in the patient's record (compared to 84 per cent of those who did report).[148] As many as 54 per cent dislike regional review committees asking for additional information.[149] Den Hartogh, a member of one of the regional review committees, confirms that his committee is frequently confronted with cross responses by euthanizing physicians when it requests additional information because the initial report was grossly inadequate. One physician responded: 'If this is how the committee views its task, I am going to think twice about reporting any future cases.'[150]

The Human Rights Committee of the United Nations has voiced concern about the low rate of reporting as well as the fact that the regional review committees almost always concluded that the physicians involved acted in accordance with the requirements of due care.[151] In response, the Dutch government has argued that the very low frequency of condemnatory judgements could also mean that the physicians involved were simply extremely meticulous and conscientious. Other proponents of the Dutch approach have remarked that euthanasia also happens abroad, but there the reporting incidence is far smaller. At least, in the Netherlands there is some control and quality improvement. But Den Hartogh has pointed out that this reply is hardly convincing. For the question remains whether the Dutch procedures really result in a different euthanasia practice. Den Hartogh has speculated that physicians only cooperate with the authorities if the official process of evaluation will not require any changes in their way of practice. As soon as this process would require changes, they will simply not report.[152] Indeed, the 1995 survey by Van der Wal showed that there is a significant difference in willingness to report between physicians who practise euthanasia most often (i.e. four or more cases in 1994–5) and those who had three or fewer cases in 1994–5. Even though the first group should have most experience with the evaluative process and be most aware of the importance and benefits of reporting, only 15 per cent reported every case compared to approximately 60 per cent of the second group.[153]

Regional Review Committees for Euthanasia

Since November 1998, cases of euthanasia and PAS are evaluated retrospectively by one of five Regional Review Committees for Euthanasia (Regionale Toetsingscommissies Euthanasie). They have continued to function after the new law legalizing euthanasia and PAS took effect in April 2002. The only difference is that a positive verdict by the committee automatically means that the physician acted legally and shall not be prosecuted. Before April 2002, a physician could still be prosecuted after such a positive evaluation by the committee. However, in practice this rarely happened. Between November 1998 and December 2001, the combined committees passed a negative evaluation only seven times (out of 6742 cases), judging that the euthanizing physicians had failed to abide by the requirements of due care. In the majority of these cases the prosecutors dismissed anyway.[154] One can therefore reasonably assume that the new law will bring about no change in the evaluation of the Dutch euthanasia practice.

A physician who commits euthanasia or assists in the patient's suicide must report his actions to the local coroner, using a preprinted form. The coroner likewise completes a preprinted form about the case and forwards all documents on to the appropriate committee. There are five of these committees (located at the offices of the five Regional Inspectorates for Health Care). Each committee consists of three voting members: a lawyer who presides, a physician and an ethicist, and three substitute members representing the same disciplines. The fourth non-voting member is again a lawyer who serves as secretary. The secretary reviews each incoming case, prepares a draft evaluation, and sends this draft together with the complete record to the other committee members. Once every three to four weeks, the committee convenes to discuss and evaluate all cases. The committee may postpone its judgement until it has received additional information from the attending physician in writing or in person.

If the committee believes that the physician has abided by all the requirements of due care, it will so inform the physician and the case is closed. If the committee believes the physician has not abided by the requirements of due care, it will not issue such a negative judgement unless and until the attending physician has been informed of this impending judgement and been given the opportunity to clarify his case. Furthermore, the committee must first share its tentative judgement with the substitute members, as well as the presidents of the other four regional committees. Note that these extra steps are not necessary if the committee thinks the physician has acted with due care.

If the committee after these additional steps still believes the physician failed to abide by the requirements of due care, this negative judgement is passed on to the office of the Joint Prosecutors General. They evaluate the case and decide to either dismiss or refer the case to the appropriate pro-secutor. This prosecutor then examines the case in greater detail and decides to either dismiss or bring the case to court.

This evaluative process appears very thorough with many levels of assessment. However, upon closer inspection the process is actually rather superficial and biased in favour of the euthanizing physician. Consider, first that the only significant source of information is the physician who euthanized the patient or assisted in her suicide. The physician is supposed to consult with at least one independent physician, and this physician is supposed to assess the patient's condition and write a report. However, this report, to be added to the patient's medical record, is frequently very short, as short as two lines.[155] Then there is the coroner. He too must submit a form to the committee, but the model form is only one page in length and does not cover the condition of the patient but only the cause of death.

Once these documents reach the committee, the secretary composes a draft assessment. In and of itself, this would seem a useful practice, provided each committee member personally analyses the full record, and the committee as a whole discusses and evaluates each case in great detail, rather than relying on the draft from the secretary. In theory this happens, but does it happen in practice as well? As mentioned, there are five committees. In 2002, each committee evaluated between 209 and 528 cases. This means that each committee member had to read and assess approximately ten dossiers per week. However, committee members presently are not reimbursed for such preparatory time (only for the time spent attending the committee meetings once every three to four weeks). This lack of compensation is an obvious disincentive for extremely busy lawyers, physicians and ethics professors to carefully read each of more than 30 case reports tabled for the upcoming meeting. Although the committee members may do so anyway, the fact remains that the Dutch government apparently is not very eager to make sure they do. The committee itself meets about 12 to 15 times per year for about two to three hours each time. A quick calculation reveals that on average each case of euthanasia/PAS is evaluated in about five minutes. Since some cases are much more complex than others and demand much more time, many other cases must be evaluated in less than a minute. In this short time, the committee must answer very difficult questions such as whether the patient's request was truly free, persistent and deliberate; whether the patient's suffering was unbearable; whether there were reasonable alternative means to relieve the patient's suffering.

These numbers raise questions about the thoroughness of the evaluations by the regional review committees. Given that 99.7 per cent of the cases were evaluated favourably, we can only conclude that the committees give physicians the benefit of the doubt in almost all instances. Note, furthermore, that the committee is required to consult all of its own members, the presidents of all other committees, and the physician himself *only* if it believes that the physician did *not* abide by the requirements of due care. If the committee believes that the physician did act with due care, he is given the benefit of the doubt and no additional verification of the committee's evaluation has to take place.

The evident bias in favour of physicians notwithstanding, one commentator has argued that a special fund should be established for those physicians who are not evaluated favourably by the committees and need legal counsel to defend themselves if they are prosecuted for murder. For every death certificate completed, a small charge should be levied to stock this fund.[156]

Errors and malpractice

If we look at the 12 instances between November 1998 and the end of 2002 in which the regional committees concluded that the physicians involved had *not* abided by the requirements of due care, we find the following. In seven of these cases (three in 1999 and four in 2002) the committee was not convinced that the consultant had been sufficiently independent. In two cases (both in 2002) the physician who committed euthanasia was not the attending physician, as the new law requires. Both are important grounds to find against a physician, but both are purely formal grounds that can be assessed relatively easily. It is far more difficult to assess whether the patient's suffering had become unbearable indeed and the request for euthanasia was authentic and persistent.

In one of the remaining cases that occurred in 2000, the physician supplied the patient with the requested lethal drugs but then left the patient, as the patient had requested. The committee nevertheless deemed that the physician should have stayed with the patient. The second case in 2000 also concerned PAS. The physician delivered the lethal drugs and, as agreed, returned two hours later. The patient's breathing did cease and the coroner was called. But 15 minutes later, the patient began to breathe again. The physician rushed to the pharmacist for advice, and in the meantime the coroner arrived to find the patient alive. Soon thereafter the patient died. In the third case in 2000, the physician and consultant believed there were quite reasonable alternatives, but the physician gave in to the insistence of the patient, therein supported by the family. The only case in 2001 in which a physician was deemed not to have abided by the requirements of due care concerned a physician who was not the attending physician of the patient, but only the patient's friend.

This overall very positive assessment is not shared by all. Ten per cent of the physicians who were surveyed by Van der Wal in 1995 were not satisfied with the way in which euthanasia/PAS had been executed. A recent reassessment of these same 1995 data led the researchers to conclude that in 3 per cent of all euthanasia cases (or almost 100 cases) there were complications such as myoclonus or vomiting. In 6 per cent or almost 200 instances, it took the patient much longer to die than expected. These problems are even more common in PAS (7 per cent and 16 per cent respectively).[157] Some physicians have publicly admitted their inability to procure a truly 'good' death. One physician wrote: 'In two or three of the eight cases of euthanasia I have performed, there were some difficult moments. In one instance after drinking the potion, a woman began to cough violently before I was able to calm her and she slipped into unconsciousness. In another instance, a patient vomited just after swallowing the drug. . . . I believe physicians ought to cooperate with veterinarians because they are far ahead of us in this area.'[158]

Why physicians?

In the preceding sections, we have focused almost exclusively on physicians and their involvement in MPD. Even though the Dutch definition of euthanasia does not include a reference to a physician, de facto almost all Dutch cases of MPD are executed by physicians. Van Wijmen found that in 1985, 89 per cent of the responding physicians believed euthanasia was the prerogative of physicians.[159] Ten years later, about the same number of physicians (87 per cent) believed that nurses should never be allowed to practise euthanasia.[160] Although a small minority (10 per cent) believe nurses can do it at the explicit instruction of a physician, none of the physicians in 1995 would allow nurses to practise euthanasia independently. The belief that only physicians can practise euthanasia is widely shared outside the medical profession (89 per cent of coroners and 90 per cent of prosecutors).

The question arises as to why physicians have agreed to shoulder the Dutch euthanasia practice; why they have insisted that other health-care providers such as nurses and pharmacists, may not practise euthanasia; and why society has readily granted physicians this monopoly? The Dutch government has stated repeatedly that euthanasia is not a *normal* medical intervention such as the administration of effective pain medications. If euthanasia would be *normal* medical practice, physicians would be obligated to perform it. Physicians have a professional obligation to perform interventions that qualify as normal medical practice. A surgeon who is also a Jehovah's Witness may not refuse to administer blood or blood products. However, the government has always insisted that physicians are not required to commit euthanasia or PAS.[161] Even though euthanasia is not a *normal* medical intervention, according to the Dutch government it is a *medical* intervention nevertheless.[162] What justifies this unusual label – *medical, though not normal medical* practice? – unusual because there appears to be no other intervention that fits this label.

It is not simply an intervention by a physician, for that would invoke a logical circle: Only physicians may practise euthanasia because euthanasia is a medical intervention; and euthanasia is a medical intervention because it is practised by physicians. The mere fact that the physician is competent to perform this intervention does not render it a medical intervention either. The undeniable competence of Dr Harold Shipman of Great Britain to commit murder does not prove mass murder is a medical intervention. Moreover, physicians certainly are not the only ones competent to perform euthanasia. Even if we were to grant that medical expertise is required to assess the need for euthanasia, the execution itself certainly does not require much medical expertise. Most nurses would be competent, as would pharmacists. Indeed, several Dutch courts have confirmed this hypothesis by requiring merely that a physician be *involved* in the process towards euthanasia.[163] Nevertheless, euthanasia is explicitly reserved for physicians by the new Dutch law.

Remarkably, the answer to this question remains forthcoming.[164] An examination of the more than one thousand pages of transcripts from parliamentary debates preceding the new law provides no convincing argument. In fact, the issue is not discussed at all. It is simply assumed that euthanasia is a medical intervention, the prerogative of physicians. Without much ado, physicians have been lifted above the law that governs all other Dutch citizens, lay people and health-care providers alike. Ending another person's life, even at that person's own request, has remained a crime, punishable with up to 12 years' imprisonment – unless one is a physician.

4 | The response of the law

Introduction

On 10 April 2001, the Netherlands became the first country to legalize euthanasia. Although the state authorities – both the attorney general's office and the independent courts – had tolerated the practice of euthanasia for several decades, it had always remained subject to legal control. For the first time in modern history it has become possible for physicians to euthanize their patients without having to defend their actions to the judiciary.

Under the new law that has taken effect in April 2002, the physician who practises euthanasia must abide by a number of specified requirements and can be prosecuted if (s)he fails to do so. For example, the patient's medical condition must be without prospect and the patient must request euthanasia. But such similar requirements apply to other normal medical interventions. For example, a surgeon acts recklessly if she embarks on a dangerous operation when less dangerous treatments are also available. Should harm come to the patient as a result, the surgeon can be prosecuted. The same is true if a physician begins antibiotic treatment without the patient's consent. Except for medical emergencies, patients must ask for help and explicitly agree with proposed treatments before the physician may initiate treatment.

In other words, the fact that a euthanizing physician must abide by these requirements of due care is nothing special. Any physician undertaking any kind of treatment has to abide by such requirements. The novelty of the new law lies in the fact that euthanasia itself, the act of terminating a patient's life, has become lawful behaviour that is sanctioned rather than prohibited by the state. Nobody in the Netherlands is allowed to end another person's life, not even at his or her own and explicit request. Anyone who does so anyway is liable to 12 years' imprisonment, except for physicians.

In this chapter, we will review how physicians acquired this remarkable legally sanctioned power. We begin with a short description of the applicable laws prior to 2002, containing clear prohibitions against euthanasia and physician assisted suicide (PAS). We then review the history of Dutch jurisprudence in the latter half of the twentieth century and show that prosecutors and courts became ever more lenient. This review will also demonstrate the peculiar reverence the Dutch legal system has for physicians compared to lay people who commit euthanasia or even other health-care providers. Not a single physician has ever been sent to jail for committing euthanasia or even ending a patient's life without the latter's request. This also raises the question why a new law, legalizing euthanasia and PAS altogether, was at all necessary, which question we will address in the final section of this chapter.

The relevance of the Dutch legal developments for other countries

It has often been said, in particular by Dutch proponents of legalized euthanasia and PAS, that the country's legal situation is so unique that euthanasia can never become an export product.[165] Granted, there are peculiarities in the Dutch Penal Code that are not found in other criminal codes. A notable example is the various articles specifying the conditions under which someone who commits a crime nevertheless is not liable to punishment. Article 40 (defining *force majeure*) is one of these articles and has played a major role in euthanasia jurisprudence (see pp. 96–9). However, we will show that this article at best provided a door through which euthanasia could be slipped into the legal system. If it had not been for this door, another one would have been found. Indeed, several other doors were tried. Once euthanasia was in the door, Article 40 quickly lost its jurisprudential significance for the practice of euthanasia. Instead, the 'prevailing standards of medical practice and medical ethics' became the guiding principle, which clearly is not a legal principle.

The manner in which euthanasia will be manoeuvred into the legal system will differ in each country. For example, in the United States with its common law tradition and its strong emphasis on civil liberties, proponents of PAS have tried to argue by analogy from a right to refuse life-sustaining treatment to a right to physician assistance in suicide. In 1997, the US Supreme Court rejected the analogy, although it also found that neither prohibition nor legalization of PAS is necessarily unconstitutional. Hence states can continue to prohibit it, or legalize it as the state of Oregon has done.

While the legal strategy to get to legalization may differ in different countries, it tends to be driven by a similar agenda. All who are interested in or concerned about legalization of euthanasia, whether Dutch or foreign, can therefore learn important lessons from the manner in which the Dutch legal system has struggled for three decades with the euthanasia movement. We will show that the Dutch legal system has neither been an effective means of preventing the practice of euthanasia and PAS, nor an effective regulator once euthanasia and PAS were decriminalized. We have no reason to believe that the legal systems in other countries will be more effective.

The law of 1886

The last major overhaul of the Dutch Penal Code occurred in 1886. Towards the end of the nineteenth century, the old French Code Pénal from 1811 was still in force even though the Netherlands had gained its independence back in 1813. King William III in 1870 ordered the development of a new Penal Code written in the Dutch language. It was completed in 1886.[166] In the section on 'crimes against life', various forms of homicide such as murder and manslaughter were defined. The act of euthanasia was not included as such, but according to Article 293 any person who kills another human person at the latter's explicit and voluntary request is liable to 12 years' imprisonment.

It is important to emphasize that the request, even if it is the explicit, persistent and urgent request of a competent and rational person, does not make the killing lawful. Because of the request, homicide at the victim's own request is not an assault against the victim himself. But the 1886 legislature argued that such homicides are still crimes against human life in general and should hence be punished. Thus the mere fact that a terminally ill patient begs her physician to end her life in and of itself does not justify the physician's actions. It only proves that the physician is not guilty of murder (as specified in Article 289 of the Penal Code) but of 'homicide at the victim's request' (as specified in Article 293), and hence is liable to 12 years' imprisonment instead of 20.

As is true of most countries, at one point in time the Netherlands also forbade suicide and imposed punishments. But neither the old French Code Pénal from 1811 nor the new Dutch Penal Code from 1886 prohibits suicide. This does not mean the Dutch state sanctions suicide. The state continues to have an interest in human life and would like to prevent suicides. However, criminalizing suicide is not an effective means of preventing suicide. One can easily see that a patient who is desperate enough to contemplate suicide will not be deterred from suicide by the threat of legal penalties. In fact, the threat of legal penalties may result in more rather than fewer suicides. Why?

One has to remember that if suicide is a crime, so is attempted suicide. All attempted crimes are criminal acts and punishable under the law. Many people who attempt suicide do so not because they actually want to die but as an ultimate cry for help. Consequently, many patients (un)consciously commit suicide in such a manner that they are likely to be found in time or use means that are somewhat likely to fail. If they are indeed found and rescued, they would now be guilty of the crime of attempted suicide and face imprisonment or other penalties. Evidently, this foresight may cause many suicidal patients to use means that 'guarantee success', resulting in more rather than fewer deaths.

These pragmatic considerations caused most countries to decriminalize suicide, including the Netherlands. However, the same considerations do not hold true for the act of assisting in suicide. Unlike the suicidal patient himself, the person who assists in the suicide is probably deterred by the threat of imprisonment or other legal penalties. By prohibiting assistance in suicide, the number of successful suicides is thought to decrease. Hence, the fact that the Dutch Penal Code from 1886 does not prohibit suicide yet prohibits assistance in suicide (Article 294) makes perfect sense and is not inconsistent (Figure 4.1).

Figure 4.1   Dutch Penal Code of 1886

Dutch Penal Code of 1886

Article 293: A person who terminates the life of another person at that other person's express and earnest request is liable to a term of imprisonment of not more than twelve years or a fine of the fifth category.

Article 294: A person who intentionally incites another to commit suicide, assist him therein, or provides the means thereto, is liable to imprisonment of not more than three years or a fine of the fourth category, where the suicide ensues.

It should be pointed out that neither Article 293 (which prohibits homicide at the victim's own request) nor Article 294 (assistance in suicide) allows for exceptions. For example, it does not matter what the offender's motive is. Indeed, the Explanatory Note that accompanied the Proposal of Law in 1886 specifically stated that the motives of the offender are irrelevant. Whether the offender acted out of anger or love, greed or mercy does not matter.[167] Likewise the status of the victim is not qualified. Killing a young person at her request is no less of a crime than killing an old person;

assisting in the suicide of a healthy person is no less a crime than assisting in the suicide of a disabled person. No exceptions are made for the status of the offender either. A lover killing his fiancée at her request would be as much guilty as a father his son or a physician her patient. And finally, no exceptions are made for the manner in which a person's life is ended. Whether he is shot through the head five times or killed with a single injection is irrelevant. The nature of the execution may impact the severity of the imposed punishment, but not the nature of the crime nor the guilt of the offender.

Even though the 1886 legislature clearly intended Articles 293 and 294 to be all-encompassing, when the first euthanasia cases surfaced a century later, several proponents of legalized euthanasia tried to argue that the legal prohibitions from 1886 simply did not apply to euthanasia cases. The drafters of the 1886 law, so the proponents argued, had never intended these articles to apply to the practice of euthanasia. Hence they had never given the example of euthanasia. They had only mentioned duels and 'Romeo-and-Juliet' type scenarios such as the one from 1859 in which a young couple, unable to marry, decided to commit suicide; she died but he did not and was then sentenced to be hanged (though on appeal acquitted).

The first court to accept this defence of euthanasia was the District Court of Alkmaar in the euthanasia case of Dr Schoonheim (for details, see pp. 100–3). In its 1983 verdict, the court first acknowledged that more and more people support the patient's right to autonomy even in regard to the termination of life. Second, that it is a well-known fact that in order to be able to end one's life in an acceptable and non-violent manner, assistance of a third party is often necessary. The court reasoned that if someone assists in ending someone else's life at that person's voluntary request, even though such an act formally constitutes a violation of Article 293 or 294, the 'material illegality' may be absent, if and only insofar as such an action from a legal perspective cannot be considered undesirable. The court then concluded that euthanasia legally was not undesirable. In other words, Articles 293 and/or 294 simply do not apply to the practice of euthanasia.

The prosecutor appealed against the verdict. The High Court of Amsterdam, dealing with the Schoonheim case on appeal, did not accept the argumentation of the District Court. The Attorney General for the High Court stated that it is not up to the judge to define the legal status of particular actions. This is the task of the legislature, and it has defined killing, including killing at the victim's request, as a crime. The fact that euthanasia was not mentioned does not necessarily mean parliament in 1886 was not concerned with the practice of physicians or even overlooked the issue altogether. In other areas of criminal law, such as abortion and surgery more in general, parliament had specifically addressed physicians and medical practice and made exceptions.

The Attorney General granted that conflicts could occur between law and medical science such that medical science should take precedence. This had happened half a century earlier. A veterinarian doctor had brought healthy cattle in contact with ill cattle in hopes of immunizing the former. Even though bringing healthy cattle in contact with ill ones formally constituted an illegal act, the case against the veterinarian had been dismissed because his actions were medically indicated and consistent with the science of veterinarian medicine. That line of reasoning could certainly be invoked analogously to justify good end-of-life care, including potentially lethal doses of analgesics that are needed to relieve the patient's pain. But the same line of reasoning does not apply to euthanasia because euthanasia is never 'medically indicated' or even 'consistent with the science of medicine'. The High Court agreed with the Attorney General.

Articles 293 and 294 of the Penal Code from 1886 did not make an exception for physicians, and if no such exception could now be created for physicians practising euthanasia, how then could it happen that no Dutch physician has ever been sent to jail for euthanizing a patient? This brings us to another part of the criminal law.

Force majeure

The Dutch Penal Code contains several articles intended to assure that justice is also done when a rigorous application of the prohibitions in the Code would lead to injustice. Literally, these are called 'punishment exclusion grounds'. They take away the liability to punishment of someone who formally has violated the law. Consider, for example, a chauffeur who tries to bypass a traffic jam by driving in the emergency lane. This chauffeur trespasses the law that prohibits such driving in emergency lanes and is therefore liable to punishment. What if the chauffeur is actually directed to drive in the emergency lane by a police officer? He would still be violating the same law that prohibits driving in emergency lanes. But surely it would be unjust to fine him when all he did was follow police instructions. Indeed, Article 43, § 1 of the Dutch Penal Code addresses this problem. It states that anyone who is directed by legal authorities to behave in a manner that would otherwise be illegal, is not liable to punishment. His actions were lawful.

But what if the police officer in reality was not a police officer. In that case, the chauffeur's behaviour could not be qualified as 'lawful' anymore. After all, there was no police officer who is authorized to temporarily direct traffic into the emergency lane. Still, it would be unfair to punish the driver who, in good faith, followed the orders from a person he honestly believed to be a genuine police officer. Indeed, Article 43, § 2 determines that this driver would not be liable to punishment either.

Another set of 'punishment exclusion grounds' concerns self-defence.

Consider a woman being attacked by a pickpocket. While defending herself she seriously harms the attacker. She would not be guilty of battery even though her actions formally constitute battery. Her battering the pick-pocket in self-defence would be lawful (Article 41, § 1). Even if the woman panicked and shot her attacker, she would not be liable to punishment (Article 42, § 2). Her excessive self-defence would itself not be justified, but she would not be blameworthy and hence not be punished. In other words, there are two different grounds why someone who formally has violated the Penal Code nevertheless is not liable to punishment. One is that the behaviour of the offender was actually just and lawful. The other is that the behaviour itself is unlawful, but the offender cannot personally be blamed and hence may not be punished.

Of course, a physician who euthanizes a patient cannot appeal to any of the punishment exclusion grounds discussed above. The physician does not act out of self-defence nor on the orders of a legal authority. However, there is one article in the Penal Code that applies generically to any and all situations in which someone feels compelled to violate the Penal Code. Article 40 states that he who commits a crime while compelled to do so by *overmacht* is not liable to punishment. The Dutch term *overmacht* literally means 'overpower' and is more commonly translated as *force majeure*. The Penal Code does not define what exactly *force majeure* means. What kind of 'power' is so severe that it will 'overpower' the person and compel him or her to violate the criminal law? Dutch jurisprudence has answered this question as follows: *Force majeure* can be understood either as 'conflict of duties' or as 'psychological *force majeure*'.[168]

This distinction reflects the earlier distinction of two grounds for pun-ishment exclusion. If an offender wants to appeal to 'conflict of duties', he will argue that a higher duty compelled him to set aside the prohibitions in the Penal Code. In other words, he was actually justified in his actions and hence should not be punished. If an offender wants to appeal to 'psycho-logical *force majeure*', he will argue that a mental force overtook him such that he was compelled to violate the penal law. Because of this mental force, he should be neither blamed nor punished for his otherwise criminal behaviour.

How would a physician charged with euthanasia successfully appeal to Article 40? Again, the two aforementioned interpretations of Article 40 can be used.[169] Let us first examine 'psychological *force majeure*'. It is impor-tant to emphasize that the offender cannot merely argue that at the moment of his deed he was mentally *different* from all other people (i.e. insane or feebleminded) and hence could not have acted otherwise. The offender has to make plausible that under similar circumstances other people might have acted similarly. One way to make such an argument is to show that it is understandable that the stressful circumstances of the case psychologically compelled the offender to act as he did (as in the pickpocket example).

Consequently, it is reasonable to presume that other people might have acted similarly under similar circumstances.

Physicians committing euthanasia have tried to make such an argument, but unsuccessfully. A euthanizing physician would have to argue (a) that he could not withstand the pressures of the situation, 'caved in' and committed euthanasia; (b) that other physicians under similar circumstances likewise would 'cave in'. But this is not a convincing line of argument. After all, physicians supposedly are able to withstand the difficult situations that arise when patients fail to recover, suffer and are dying. That is what they are trained for, or what they should be trained for.[170]

Indeed, most proponents of euthanasia argue that physicians do not commit euthanasia because they are compelled to do so by psychological forces. Euthanasia generally is not practised by physicians who know quite well that euthanasia is morally and legally wrong, but are overpowered by the mental stresses of the situation. Rather, these physicians commit euthanasia because they think the act of euthanasia is moral and right. Therefore, not the actor but the act itself should be excused. This brings us to the other interpretation of Article 40, 'conflict of duties'. Most physicians committing euthanasia have appealed to 'conflict of duties', and successfully so. When appealing to 'conflict of duties', the offender has to acknowledge that (a) he has a duty to act in accordance with the law; (b) he also has a duty to foster some other important interest; (c) these two duties became incompatible in the given situation; (d) having to balance the various interests at stake, most other people could have reasonably chosen to protect the same interest he chose to protect, even if it meant violating the law.

Again it is important to emphasize that 'most other people' could have reasonably chosen to protect the conflicting interest. Personal conscience typically is not shared by 'most other people' and cannot be verified. In 1952, the District Court of Utrecht was the first to face a euthanasia case. It concerned a physician who had euthanized his own brother by administering 18 to 20 capsules of 10 mg codinovo tablets, followed by an injection of 60 mg of morphine. The patient was suffering severely from tuberculosis. The physician argued that his own conscience had forced him to end his brother's life. But the court objected that Dutch law does not allow for such an appeal in euthanasia cases (as it does in cases of military draft or compulsory vaccinations). The District Court of Utrecht rejected the appeal and imposed a probationary sentence of one year's imprisonment.

The question thus arises as to what duty exactly forces physicians to commit euthanasia. What medical duty is so urgent that it can take priority over the medical-ethical and legal obligation not to kill another human being, not even at his or her own request? As we have seen, even the Dutch legislature of 1886 did not believe there was such a duty. It is the answer to this most fundamental of questions that legally distinguishes the

Netherlands from virtually all other countries. And in order to answer it, we have to turn to Dutch jurisprudence.[171]

Jurisprudential developments

The 1973 verdict of the District Court of Leeuwarden in the Postma case revisited

The earliest case in which a euthanizing physician appealed to Article 40 occurred in the early 1970s. It was only the second euthanasia case recorded in Dutch jurisprudence (the first was in 1952). As described in Chapter 1. (pp. 5–6) Dr Postma had ended the life of her 78-year-old mother with a single injection of 200 mg of morphine. Her mother had been paralysed on one side of her body, incontinent, and suffering from pneumonia. She was restless, resulting in the use of restraints, at times aggressive, and unwilling to cooperate with rehabilitation attempts. Instead, she repeatedly voiced a wish for her life to be ended.

The District Court of Leeuwarden rejected the physician's appeal to Article 40 because it had become evident that ending the patient's life was not the only means left to relieve the patient's suffering. Other reasonable alternatives had been available, including high doses of psychoactive palliative medications. According to the court, administering such drugs that are known to shorten a patient's life is not illegal, provided they are administered for the sole purpose of relieving pain. But administering a lethal dosage of drugs in order to end the patient's life is illegal. The court decided that Dr Postma should at least have tried these alternative and legal means first.

Proponents of euthanasia hailed the court's decision to impose a probationary sentence of one week only. But the actual verdict would suggest that if a physician does not use alternative means available, she certainly cannot be in a conflict of duties. The court listed both high doses of palliative medications (morphine and/or psychoactive drugs), as well as forgoing life-sustaining treatment as alternatives to be tried first. Since both options are open in virtually any and all cases, it was unclear whether a euthanizing physician could ever successfully appeal to Article 40.

The 1981 verdict of the District Court of Rotterdam in the Wertheim case

In 1981, the District Court of Rotterdam was faced with Mrs Wertheim who had assisted in the suicide of her friend. The defence attorney acknowledged that assistance in suicide had been added to the 1886 Penal

Code because the legislature wanted to prevent suicides. However, times had changed and so had the public's opinion about suicide. The court agreed that in exceptional cases suicide was not immoral and assisting in such a suicide, hence, should not be viewed as a crime either. In such circumstances, the physician would not be liable to punishment.

The court listed a series of conditions (see Table 4.1) which, taken together, defined an exceptional case. Among them were the requirement that the patient's suffering was long-lasting and unbearable and, again, that there were no alternatives to relieve the suffering. In addition, it listed a number of prudential requirements concerning the actual performance of euthanasia in such exceptional cases, such as the requirement that a physician is involved and the decision is never reached by one person only.

In this particular case, a number of the requirements set by the court had not been met. Among others, the offender was not a physician and had acted hastily. Moreover, it remained unclear whether the patient's desire to die was really lasting and all reasonable alternatives for 'meaningful palliative care' had been depleted. The court therefore rejected the appeal to Article 40, but the door to legally sanctioned euthanasia had been opened. The requirements listed by the District Court of Rotterdam suggested that a euthanizing physician might be able to successfully appeal to Article 40. This happened two years later.

The 1983 verdict of the District Case of Alkmaar in the Schoonheim case

Mrs S, born in 1886, had been a patient of Dr Schoonheim since 1974. As her family physician, he had seen her many times, on some of which occasions Mrs S had asked him whether it was possible to end her life by means of a medical procedure. One day Mrs S presented Dr Schoonheim with a euthanasia testament, which he accepted.

Despite her age, mentally Mrs S remained in very good condition, but physically she declined rapidly. Then she broke her hip. Since an operation was not possible, she was confined to her bed. She suffered gravely as her physical condition worsened visibly. Her requests for ending her life became more frequent and urgent. In early July 1982, the patient's condition suddenly deteriorated. She was unable to eat or drink and lost consciousness. On 12 July, she regained consciousness and told Dr Schoonheim that never again did she want to go through another such breakdown. Once more, she asked to be killed. When finally Mrs S's son begged him to fulfill his mother's wishes, Dr Schoonheim decided to honour her request.

On 16 July 1982, at 11:00 am, Dr Schoonheim had a final discussion with his patient. Present were her son and his wife as well as Dr

Schoonheim's assistant, Dr B. Once again, Mrs S conveyed that she had just one wish left: to die as soon as possible. With three consecutive injections that put Mrs S to sleep, then into a coma and finally stopped her breathing, Dr Schoonheim fulfilled the last wish of his patient.

On 10 May 1983, the District Court of Alkmaar issued its verdict. As pointed out earlier (see p. 95), the defence attorney initially maintained that Articles 293 and 294 simply do not pertain to the practice of euthanasia. This argument was accepted by the Alkmaar Court, resulting in a dismissal.

Table 4.1 Requirements of due care

	Leeuwarden 1973	Rotterdam 1981	Alkmaar 1983	Groningen 1984
Condition of the patient				
Incurably diseased	Y		Y	Y
Suffering is • long-lasting		Y	Y	
• somatic				
• somatic or mental	Y	Y		
• unbearable		Y	Y	Y
• serious or unbearable	Y			
In the dying phase				
Hopeless situation				
No other reasonable solution	Y	Y		
Request				
By patient himself	Y	Y	Y	Y
Only by adult patient				
No hidden signal for help		Y	Y	
Voluntary		Y	Y	
Deliberate		Y	Y	Y
Repeated or lasting		Y	Y	
Practice				
By physician				Y
After patient counselling				
Consultation by • State appointed MD				
• independent physician				
• some other MD	Y	Y	Y	
• relevant expert				
MD logbook of history				
Third persons				
Consultation of family			Y	
No unnecessary harm results for others		Y		

But it was rejected on appeal by the High Court of Amsterdam. The High Court furthermore argued that Article 40 could not be invoked either. It was not convinced that the suffering of the patient was so unbearable that Dr Schoonheim had had no option left but to end the life of the patient. It concluded that Dr Schoonheim was liable to punishment (which, strangely, the High Court then did not impose, not even a probationary sentence).

The case was appealed once more to the Supreme Court. It argued that the High Court of Amsterdam had adequately established that Article 40 could not be invoked *when interpreted as psychological force majeure*. Dr Schoonheim was not under such severe psychological pressures that he *had* to commit euthanasia. However, the High Court had not adequately proven that there was no *conflict of duties*. The High Court of Amsterdam should have examined whether 'according to responsible medical opinion, corroborated by the prevailing norms of medical ethics, a conflict of interests existed'. More specifically, the High Court should have examined (a) whether a further corrosion of the personal dignity of the patient and/or a worsening of her already unbearable suffering was likely; (b) whether it would soon be impossible for the patient to die in a dignified manner as a result of her worsening condition. The Supreme Court hence nullified the verdict of the High Court of Amsterdam and referred the case to the High Court of The Hague for final adjudication.

The High Court of The Hague concluded that other means of relief, specifically psychoactive drugs, had been exhausted – even though this was only the case because the patient had refused those drugs. Next it granted that there was certainly no general consensus among Dutch physicians that euthanasia was a justifiable response to her unbearable suffering. Nevertheless, Dr Schoonheim's choice for euthanasia was justified according to medical-ethical standards. The High Court accepted the appeal to Article 40 and concluded that Dr Schoonheim was not liable to punishment.

This first verdict by the Dutch Supreme Court in a euthanasia case seems to provide an answer to our crucial question: What medical duty is so urgent that it can take priority over the legal obligation not to kill another human being, not even at his or her own request? The Supreme Court appears to reason that a physician may have the duty to end a patient's life (at her request) if there is a severe corrosion of human dignity and/or unbearable suffering that cannot be relieved by other means. But is life ever so undignified that a physician can justifiably kill the patient? If so, who determines whether that point has been reached?

Note that it cannot simply be left up to the patient to make that determination. In that case, the determination of the unbearableness of suffering would collapse into the patient's request. All the patient would have to do is say that her life is unbearable and that she therefore wants euthanasia. Furthermore, we have seen before that the request of the patient only changes the act from plain murder into homicide at the victim's request.

The request itself cannot possibly justify ending the patient's life; such requested homicide remains an affront against human life and hence a criminal act.

If not the patient, then who determines whether the patient's life has indeed become undignified or her suffering unbearable? The Supreme Court answered that it must be examined whether 'according to responsible medical opinion, corroborated by the prevailing norms of medical ethics, a conflict of interests existed'. We do not know whether in 1984 the Supreme Court was fully aware of the lasting and decisive impact of these words. In hindsight we can see that this single sentence set the stage for all future jurisprudence on euthanasia cases, as well as the new law from 2001. The court's failure to give a substantive answer, referring instead to 'medical opinion and the prevailing norms of medical ethics', meant that the court had deferred to the medical profession, *de facto* as well as *de iure*.

Whether the Supreme Court intended that to happen in unclear. But it is certainly clear that the Supreme Court believed that physicians are much more likely to be in such a conflict of duties than lay people. Why? If anybody committing euthanasia in principle can invoke *force majeure*, but physicians are much more likely to do so successfully, what causes this exceptional immunity against legal retribution? In the Schoonheim case, the various courts said little to answer this question. But at the same time as the Schoonheim case was being decided, a new case surfaced in Groningen. The issue of the 'medical exception' became the focus of the Groningen case, the second euthanasia case to make it all the way to the Dutch Supreme Court – twice.

The 1984 verdict of the District Court of Groningen in the Pols case

One day in August 1982, Dr Pols, a psychiatrist in the Dutch province of Groningen, informed the prosecutor that she had committed euthanasia on Mrs M. The physician had been a good friend of Mrs M, a 73-year-old lady with multiple sclerosis. When they had first met, Mrs M had suffered a major deterioration of her physical situation and started talking about euthanasia. She had lived a difficult life, but had always fought back and managed to regain control over the situation. This time, fighting seemed utterly useless. Not being able to change the course of her disease, she refused any of the alternative medications Dr Pols proposed.

Sometime in the middle of 1982, Dr Pols started making preparations for euthanasia. She contacted various physicians and met with a pastor. With an anaesthetist and a pharmacist, she discussed the best technique. Dr Pols checked again with Mrs M whether she still wanted to die. Finally, on 4 August, Dr Pols gave her friend seconal and a glass of port wine. Mrs M started talking nonsense and then lost consciousness. Two hours later, Mrs M had still not died. Being afraid that one of the nursing home personnel might pass by and start resuscitation, Dr Pols injected morphine. She then delivered a letter to the prosecutor to inform him about her actions.

On 1 March 1984, the District Court of Groningen found that Dr Pols could neither invoke 'psychological *force majeure*' nor 'conflict of duties'. It concluded that the interest which the law intends to protect with Article 293 (i.e. human life) can never be superseded by the alleged goals of euthanasia. This sweeping conclusion seemed to slam the door shut on any and all appeals by euthanizing physicians to Article 40.

However, the Groningen Court came up with a new line of argument. If somebody has been found guilty of committing a crime, it is nevertheless possible to find him *not* liable to punishment, if such a deed is

• a medical intervention;
• necessary for medical reasons or of critical importance for adequate medical care;
• and all due care is applied that medical science and practice require.

It will be clear that these three conditions presumably apply to any and all medical interventions. Earlier we saw that the Leeuwarden District Court in the Postma case had already come to similar conclusions regarding the use of potentially lethal pain medications (see p. 99; see also Chapter 1, p. 5). However, never before had euthanasia been considered a medical act proper. But the Groningen Court changed all that. It argued that someone committing euthanasia could likewise be immune to legal retribution under the following conditions:

1 The person committing euthanasia was a physician.
2 The euthanizing physician had consulted with another physician who had seen the patient.
3 Euthanasia was practised on a patient whose condition was irreversible and experienced by the patient as unbearable suffering.
4 The explicit and earnest request for euthanasia by the patient could be considered lasting and based on a proper evaluation by the patient of his own condition and the alternatives available.
5 The patient did not believe there was a reasonable alternative.
6 All other requirements for a careful and prudential execution of euthanasia had been fulfilled.

But the High Court of Leeuwarden that dealt with the case on appeal, forcefully disagreed. The mere fact that it is a physician who commits an act in accordance with the guidelines of the medical profession does not exclude the offender from punishment. The High Court granted that genuine medical interventions certainly do not fall under the criminal law. To remove an inflamed appendix, the surgeon has to cut the patient. Even though anybody else who cuts another person with a knife can be prosecuted for battery, surgeons cannot because their cutting patients falls under the so-called 'medical exception'. However, unlike surgery to remove an appendix, or even abortion to save the life of the mother, euthanasia is not *genuine* medicine. Even proponents of euthanasia generally agree that euthanasia is *not* medical practice proper. An appeal to the medical exception as a punishment exclusion ground for euthanasia therefore had to be rejected.

Dr Pols appealed. Two years later, on 21 October 1986, the Supreme Court for the second time dealt with a euthanasia case. It agreed with the High Court and rejected the physician's appeal to the medical exception. But it did not totally agree with the verdict of the High Court. As it had done in the Schoonheim case, the Supreme Court once again stated that the judges of the High Court had failed to thoroughly examine whether, 'according to scientifically responsible medical opinion and the prevailing norms of medical ethics', Dr Pols had been compelled by *force majeure*. It sent the case back to a different High Court for final adjudication.

The High Court of Arnhem was particularly perturbed by the fact that Dr Pols had been both the patient's physician and a close friend. This made it impossible for the physician to assess the situation objectively; she should have consulted another physician. Since she had not done so, she could not successfully invoke conflict of duties, which requires an objective assessment of the conflicting interests and duties involved. Thus the court deemed Dr Pols liable to punishment and imposed a probationary penalty of two months' imprisonment. But Dr Pols appealed once more and the case ended up in the Supreme Court for a second time. In 1988 the Supreme Court rejected the reasoning of the High Court of Arnhem as well. Dr Pols' failure to consult another physician does not necessarily imply that she could not invoke *force majeure*. Nevertheless, there was no *force majeure* in this case, because the patient's illness was not terminal. Moreover, the patient's condition was not on a downhill slope. Instead, she had just recovered somewhat when Dr Pols committed euthanasia. The Supreme Court rejected Dr Pols' appeal.

Why physicians?

In his official Commentary appended to the first verdict of the Supreme Court in the Groningen case involving Dr Pols, G. E. Mulder aptly noticed that on the one hand, the Supreme Court rejected the medical exception, but on the other hand introduced a new kind of medical exception, hidden behind the veil of Article 40. It is called *force majeure*, but actually it is not.

As explained, somebody making an appeal to *force majeure* as a punishment exclusion ground has to show that *anybody* else might have acted similarly under similar circumstances. But according to the Supreme Court, it is sufficient if *most other members of the medical profession* might have acted similarly. Why is it that a physician goes unpunished if *most other members of the medical profession* might have acted similarly. Because he is the only one who can judge whether the patient is incurable, whether there are alternatives and whether the request is not a hidden signal for help? But if that is the case, then the criterion of being a physician is superfluous, for the other requirements of due care already guarantee all this (see Table 4.1).

The courts' response to mercy killing by lay people

The Supreme Court's deference to the medical profession would have been less perplexing if only physicians were committing euthanasia. But as a matter of fact by 1986 Dutch courts had already been faced with several cases of mercy killing by lay people. The first euthanasia case of 1952 involved a physician, but the victim was the physician's brother. The court proceedings make clear that the physician primarily acted as the victim's brother, that is, as a lay person and not as a physician. No reference is made to the professional role and duties of medical professionals. Instead, the physician appealed to his personal conscience (which appeal was rejected by the court). The second euthanasia case from 1973 again involved a physician relative, but in this instance, the court specifically mentioned that euthanasia could only be justified if a physician was involved. Note, however, that euthanasia did not have to be *performed* by a physician; it sufficed if a physician was involved.

The next three euthanasia cases all involved non-physicians. The District Court of Rotterdam (12 January 1981) in the Wertheim case (pp. 99–100) once again argued that a physician should have been involved; likewise the High Court of Amsterdam (16 February 1982) in a case against a spouse. Ten months later, the District Court of Utrecht (21 December 1982) dealt with yet another spouse who had committed euthanasia on his wife. The prosecutor argued that the man had been imprudent by not consulting a physician.

Then came the famous 1983 Schoonheim case that involved a physician who was neither related to nor befriended the patient (see pp. 100–3). For the first time, the Supreme Court (27 November 1984) referred to the standards of medical practice and the prevailing medical-ethical norms, thereby creating a medical monopoly on euthanasia. It reinforced this monopoly two years later in the Pols case (21 November 1986) (see pp. 103–5). Of course, this was not the end to non-medical euthanasia cases. But if it ever had been easy for lay people to successfully appeal to

Article 40 – in the formerly described cases of non-medical euthanasia, one lay person was sent to jail and the other two were given probationary sentences – the Supreme Court verdicts seemed to have further reduced their chances. On 8 March 1984, the District Court of Breda imposed a probationary sentence of one year's imprisonment. On 23 July 1985, the District Court of Utrecht imposed one year's imprisonment, not probationary. So did the District Court of Alkmaar on 8 July 1986.

In 1992, the District Court of Rotterdam was again faced with a physician who was a close friend of the patient. Sure enough, the physician's appeal to conflict of duties was rejected because the physician had acted first and foremost as friend rather than as medical professional when he assisted in the patient's suicide (7 December 1992). The High Court of The Hague and the Supreme Court confirmed the lower court's verdict. Euthanasia had become a 'medical intervention' (District Court of Groningen, 26 July 1994). Maybe euthanasia was still not *normal* medical practice, but it had become the prerogative of physicians nonetheless.

Why physicians? Why is it that physicians are more likely to face a conflict of duties than a good friend, a brother or a spouse? It seems counter-intuitive that a physician's moral obligation to relieve the suffering of a dying person is greater than the moral duty of a daughter towards her dying mother. This counter-intuitive distinction makes sense only if one were to assume that the very practice of medicine generates this conflict of duties between respect for human life and relief of suffering. One would have to hypothesize that the very ethos of medical practice causes physicians to give priority to the relief of suffering over the fight for life. This line of argumentation would also make the Supreme Court's deference to the prevailing norms of medical ethics more convincing. But is this hypothesis true to the reality of medical practice?

The most obvious weakness in this line of reasoning is the evident fact that such a duty to end the lives of patients has never been subscribed to in the Netherlands prior to the early 1970s; nor was or is it subscribed to by the medical profession in any other country (except for the euthanasia practice in Nazi Germany – and even that had to be kept largely a secret, fearing opposition from both religious leaders and medical professionals). Thus, Dutch proponents of medical euthanasia would either have to argue that all the professional medical organizations elsewhere in the world have it wrong; or the health-care context in the Netherlands is so unique that Dutch medical practice cannot be compared with the practice of physicians elsewhere in the world.

The courts' response to mercy killing by nurses

Although both are rather unconvincing arguments, the second of the two at least is not a priori absurd. Maybe there is something quite peculiar and atypical about the provision of health care in the Netherlands. But if true, one can reasonably expect that other Dutch health-care professionals are likewise impacted by the unusual health-care context that allegedly exists. The one profession that comes immediately to mind is the nursing profession. Like everywhere else in the world, nurses tend to spend more time caring for terminally ill and dying patients than any other health-care professional, including physicians. So how have euthanizing nurses fared in Dutch courts?

The first case in which a nurse was guilty of mercy killing occurred in the mid-1970s. It concerned a nurse (Frans H) who had killed a number of patients without their request. In its verdict from 7 December 1976 the District Court of Maastricht imposed 12 years' imprisonment, which penalty was increased to 18 years on appeal. Though a case of mercy killing as opposed to euthanasia (because the patients had not asked to be killed), its relevance to our discussion becomes evident when we compare it to the first case in which a physician was found guilty of mercy killing.

The patient, a 93-year-old lady, had been a patient of the family physician for some 15 years. She had multiple diseases, mostly due to her old age, but was mentally still very clear. She had indicated that she did not see any purpose in continuing living, did not fear death, and rejected life-extending medical treatments. She also rejected euthanasia, believing she had to bear her complaints. The physician believed otherwise. After a hip fracture, she refused hospitalization. The physician administered morphine to relieve her pain and she slipped into a coma. The next day, after consultation with the nursing staff and the family, the physician ended her life by injecting morphine, atropine and alloferine. The District Court of Haarlem concluded that a patient's wish that life will end soon does not equate an explicit request for euthanasia. It also rejected the physician's appeal to Article 40. Though guilty of murder, the District Court imposed a probationary sentence of one week only (4 April 1986).

One year later, the District Court of Rotterdam was faced again with a nurse who had ended the life of a patient by suffocating her. The patient was 21 years old, the last 18 of which he had lived in a mental institution. He was seriously ill, unable to walk, barely able to communicate, and tube fed. More importantly, the patient was not cared for properly. Adequate pain treatment was being withheld, so the nurse contended. This had forced him into a conflict of duties such that he was compelled to euthanize the patient. But on 31 March 1987 the court rejected the nurse's appeal to 'conflict of duties', arguing that nurses have a duty to protect patients' lives, but not to relieve patients' pain (unless at the order of a physician). The court imposed 12 months' imprisonment of which seven months were probationary. (On appeal, the High Court reduced the imprisonment to ten weeks.)

The court's assertion that only physicians have a duty to relieve patients' pain is not very convincing. Most nurses will disagree, insisting instead that they too have a duty to relieve pain and to make sure that patients do not suffer. In fact, they will argue that their duty to relieve suffering is at least as forceful as the physician's duty to do so. Nurses often view themselves as patient advocates who have to protect patients when physicians appear primarily interested in curing them. They frequently initiate discussions about forgoing life-sustaining treatment, advocating comfort care instead. In short, when a balance must be struck between protecting life and relieving suffering, it is physicians who generally claim that the duty to protect life takes priority, whereas many nurses will claim the duty to relieve suffering precedes.

On 30 March 1988 the District Court of Amsterdam reiterated the earlier verdict by the District Court of Rotterdam. It argued that euthanasia is not compatible with the science of nursing and the prevailing norms of nursing ethics. It defended its conclusion by pointing out that nurses may never administer medications at their own initiative. Hence, euthanasia cannot be part of the nurse's role. But this is a weak defence because euthanasia technically is quite simple. Moreover, the argument relies completely on the assumption that euthanasia has to be committed by administering medications.

Seven years later, the District Court of Groningen (23 March 1995) faced another case of euthanasia by a nurse. It rejected the nurse's appeal to *force majeure*, even though the nurse had consulted a physician. The court simply claimed that euthanasia is a medical intervention and the nurse should have known this. Moreover, the official guidelines – which had been accepted by the Dutch legislature in 1993 and had taken effect in 1994 – only concerned physicians. The court deduced that the legislature's failure to include nurses in the guidelines meant that nurses were intentionally excluded.

The irony of the latter argument is striking. Ten years earlier, proponents of euthanasia had argued that the very failure of the 1886 legislature to mention physicians when it drafted Articles 293 and 294 of the new Penal Code meant that these articles did not apply to physicians; hence euthanasia by physicians was lawful. The same line of reasoning now was used *against* the nursing profession: The fact that nurses were not mentioned in the new law meant that they could *not* legally practise euthanasia.

By the mid-1990s, the Dutch medical profession had managed to secure a sound legal monopoly on the practice of euthanasia. Euthanasia had become the prerogative of physicians and only physicians could judge their euthanizing colleagues. The only thing that mattered was whether euthanasia was performed in accordance with medical and medical-ethical guidelines. The courts had become fully dependent on the medical profession.

Who can speak on behalf of the medical profession?

If euthanasia was justified only when performed in accordance with 'sci-entifically responsible medical opinion and the prevailing norms of medical ethics', how could these 'objective' insights and norms be established? Would it require consensus among all Dutch physicians? Consensus among a large majority of physicians? Would a sizeable minority suffice? What was the Supreme Court thinking in 1985 when it advanced this new criterion?

The ambiguity soon became apparent when the High Court of The Hague (to which the Supreme Court had forwarded the Schoonheim case) acknowledged that a considerable number of Dutch physicians accepted euthanasia, but other Dutch physicians do not. Apparently, there was no generally accepted medical-ethical norm favouring euthanasia. Yet the High Court (10 June 1985 and 11 September 1986) decided that the choice of Dr Schoonheim had been justified by reasonable medical opinion. Almost ten years later, there was still no consensus among Dutch physicians regarding euthanasia. But the High Court of The Hague (25 May 1993) again argued that a conflict of duties can exist for a physician who assists in suicide, even if a number of Dutch physicians reject such a duty to end the life of the patient.

If consensus or even agreement among a large majority of Dutch physi-cians was not required, how then could it be assessed whether euthanasia in any given case was consistent with the standards of medical science and medical ethics? There was no option left to the courts but to rely on indi-vidual expert witnesses. So we find that time and again, medical ethicists known to favour euthanasia (such as professors Kuitert and De Beaufort) became the expert witnesses. They testified that in the case at hand euthanasia was consistent with medical-ethical guidelines, even though the debate among Dutch medical ethicists on euthanasia was ongoing and vehement with no consensus in sight.

Requirements of due care

Except for the first case of euthanasia in 1952 in which the District Court of Utrecht rejected euthanasia outright, ever since the 1970s Dutch courts have proposed requirements that must be met for euthanasia to be justified. They used these requirements to judge the offenders. In most early cases, the courts concluded that these requirements had not been fulfilled, leaving the offenders liable to punishment. But at the same time, their definition of these requirements opened the door for lawful euthanasia. The obvious implication was that if only the physician had met those requirements, (s)he would not have been liable to punishment.

Initially, the requirements were manifold and rather restrictive. But Table

4.1 shows that there was no consensus among the different courts. A closer examination of these requirements also reveals their divergent status and weight. Even though these requirements are often lumped together as 'requirements of due care', there are really three different classes of requirements.

First, there are the requirements that are already entailed in Article 293 itself which defines euthanasia. For example, the requirement that the patient should request euthanasia herself merely fulfills the description of euthanasia given in Article 293. If the patient had not asked, the physician would be guilty of 'murder' (Article 289) instead of 'homicide at the victim's request' (Article 293) and be liable to 20 instead of 12 years' imprisonment. The same is true for the requirement that the request be deliberate and consistent.

The second category of requirements specifies the conditions under which someone committing euthanasia can successfully appeal to *force majeure*. Here we find the requirement that the patient's medical condition should be without prospect of improvement. This requirement is not part of the definition of Article 293. As we saw earlier, Article 293 applies across the board to any and all people requesting to be killed. Thus, by requiring that the patient be suffering unbearably, the range of lawful euthanasia cases is significantly reduced.

The third category of requirements concerns the actual performance of euthanasia. These requirements are supposed to guarantee a prudential and technically correct euthanasia practice. Here we find the requirement that an independent physician should be involved in the decision-making process, that a log book be kept, and that no harm should come to third persons.

The fact that such very different requirements were combined into one list and that, moreover, the selection of requirements differed significantly from court to court, reveals the instability of Dutch legal thinking about euthanasia. In fact, proponents of legalized euthanasia used the confusion to argue their case. Consider for example the requirement to consult with another physician. Although such consultation was already listed early on as one of the important requirements, the High Court of The Hague (2 April 1987) did not think consultation is always necessary and neither did the Supreme Court in its decisions of 23 June 1987 and 3 May 1988. How could this happen? We must bear in mind that the crucial test for *force majeure* is whether the euthanizing physician acted in accordance with medical scientific insights and the prevailing norms of medical ethics. Whereas consultation may clarify to the physician that (s)he is indeed acting in accordance with these insights and norms, even a physician who does not consult another physician de facto may still be acting in accordance with the insights and norms. In short, failure to consult may be sloppy, but it does not necessarily affect the justification for the physician's actions.

It will be clear that this line of reasoning also holds true for physicians who commit euthanasia under the new law from 10 April 2001. Although that law once again requires consultation with another independent physician, a euthanizing physician who fails to do so can still invoke *force majeure*. The fact that he did not consult does not prove he was not compelled to act by a conflict of duties; it just makes it more difficult for the physician to prove that he was. The same thing is likely to happen with the other requirements listed in the new law. Let us therefore briefly review the three most important of these requirements: the request by the patient, the availability of alternatives, and the patient's medical condition.

The patient's request

The only criterion that has been mentioned consistently by all the courts is the request of the patient. It is listed again in the new 2001 law on euthanasia. But as early as 1988, the District Court of Almelo (1 March 1988) had found a physician liable to punishment because there had been no request from either the patient *or* the family. This raises the question as to whether the patient's own request is truly an absolute requirement. Would this physician's appeal to *force majeure* have been successful if only the family had requested termination of life? Consider the following case:

On 25 March 1993 baby Rianne was born. She had a number of very serious handicaps, including hydrocephalus, myelomeningocele, paralysis, incontinence, and severe mental retardation. Discussion with the parents led to a decision not to attempt surgical correction of the life-threatening conditions, since the prospect for a good quality of life would remain minimal anyway. But the parents insisted that Dr Prins actively end the baby's life. Three days after she was born, he did.

On 26 April 1995 the District Court of Alkmaar found the physician guilty of murder, but accepted conflict of duties. It listed four requirements, all of which the physician had met:

1 There has to be prospectless and unbearable suffering that is incurable and cannot be relieved in a medically meaningful manner.
2 There has to be the greatest possible carefulness in both reaching the decision and executing it.
3 The actions of the physician have to conform with the medical scientific insights and the prevailing norms of medical ethics.
4 Termination of life has to occur at the explicit, repeated and consistent request of the parents.

We thus find that even though the patient had not requested euthanasia, even though the physician's actions amounted to murder, the Court accepted *force majeure* and judged that the killing of baby Rianne was justified.

In the same month that the Alkmaar Court issued its verdict in the case of Dr Prins, a baby was born in a hospital in Delfzijl. Soon after her birth she was diagnosed with Trisomy 13, had several cranial deformities as well as cardiopulmonary and renal problems. Since she was expected to live only briefly, a decision was made not to resuscitate her should she suffer a cardiopulmonary arrest. The parents took the baby home, but her condition worsened so she had to be readmitted. Three weeks after her birth, the attending family physician, Dr Kadijk, ended her life at the request of the parents.

Once again, the physician was found to have committed murder, but not liable to punishment because of *force majeure* (District Court of Groningen, 13 November 1995). Then came the case of Dr van Oijen.

He was a well-known advocate of euthanasia. Like his American colleague Dr Kevorkian, he had taped one of his cases and turned it into a documentary video that was broadcast all over the world. On an early February day in 1997, he had ended the life of another patient. She had suffered for years of severe osteoporosis, forcing her to remain in bed most of the day. In turn, she developed decubitus and even necrosis. She refused physical therapy but accepted high doses of different pain medications. On 28 January Dr van Oijen had explicitly asked her whether she wanted to be 'put to sleep', which she refused. She wanted to be with her children instead. The pain medications were increased even further and when Dr van Oijen visited her on 3 February, she was lying in bed almost unconscious and in a foetal position. On 4 February he prescribed valium just in case she woke up and was restless. He expected her to die any day. But when he returned on 5 February she still had not passed away. She stank because of the necrosis. The nurse manager of the institution had given orders not to clean her anymore. Her daughters had been with her all night and they insisted that their mother would have never wanted this. Dr van Oijen indicated that she would probably die later that day, but he could also speed up her death. When the daughters chose the latter option, he administered alloferine and the patient died.

The first court to deal with this case was the Medical Disciplinary Court of Amsterdam. On 4 May 1998 it found against Dr van Oijen. Now faced with a criminal suit, he appealed against his prosecution all the way to the Supreme Court, but lost. On 21 February 2001, days before the Upper House of parliament was scheduled to vote on the new law, the District Court of Amsterdam found Dr van Oijen guilty of murder since the patient had never indicated she wanted euthanasia. On the contrary, she had expressed a wish to be with her daughters instead. The Court did not accept *force majeure* either, because the patient was simply unaware of her own condition. Hence she could not be said to be suffering unbearably. Yet no punishment was imposed, not even a probationary sentence. Two weeks later, the Upper House passed the bill legalizing euthanasia.

Ever since the empirical studies from 1990 and 1995 (discussed in Chapter 3), it has been known that a significant number of patients are killed each year by Dutch physicians without their request. If we combine this fact with the equally troublesome finding that the Dutch courts have been almost as lenient towards physicians who engaged in MPD with or without the patient's request, one can only wonder whether under the new law the courts will be any less forgiving towards physicians who kill patients without their request.

No reasonable alternatives

We have seen that the Dutch courts, beginning with the 1973 Postma case adjudicated by the District Court of Leeuwarden, have always insisted that euthanasia had to be the very last resort. As long as there were other alternatives that had not been tried, the euthanizing physician could not claim that (s)he was compelled to end the patient's life and therefore should not be punished. This would seem to be a very objective criterion. The availability of alternative treatments can be determined using sound scientific biomedical information. But a review of several court cases reveals that this important criterion could be moulded and manipulated as well.

In the former section, we reviewed the District Court of Alkmaar's 1995 decision in the case of Dr Prins and baby Rianne. The court had argued that termination of life was justifiable only if the patient's suffering was pro-spectless and unbearable and could not be relieved in any other medically meaningful manner. It is striking that the court readily accepted the view of the expert witness, Dr Versluys, that there were only two options: surgical interventions or termination of life. Versluys characterized the obvious third alternative, good palliative care while forgoing aggressive life-sustaining treatment as 'indecisive, ambiguous and likely to induce an absurd situation'.

When pressed on this point by the High Court of Amsterdam that handled the appeal, Versluys conceded that it was possible to administer high doses of painkillers, but baby Rianne would end up 'hovering between earth and heaven'. Such a situation of uncertainty would be 'exceedingly burdensome to the parents, the nurses and the attending physicians'. A second medical expert added that a palliative care approach would be medically meaningless if death was the intent, as it was in this case (or so he claimed). The High Court once again found that Dr Prins had acted in a conflict of duties and hence was not liable to punishment (7 November 1995).

Even more remarkable was the reasoning by the District Court of Groningen in the Kadijk case involving a baby with Trisomy 13 (see p. 113). During the court proceedings, the question arose once again as to whether palliative care had been possible. One of the expert witnesses argued it was, although such medications could easily cause the patient to die because of her poor renal function. Nevertheless, the District Court of Groningen accepted the assessment of another expert witness that palliative care was no longer a meaningful option.

Still stranger had been the reasoning by the District Court of Rotterdam ten years earlier in its verdict of 20 March 1985. It had concluded that there were no reasonable alternatives for symptom relief. First, further increases of morphine would have had serious medical side effects, including diminished consciousness and shortening of life. How the latter can be a serious side effect when the alternative is euthanasia remains unclear. Second, the patient had refused further increases in morphine because she wanted to retain complete consciousness.

The second argument is maybe the most troubling of all. As all competent patients, a dying patient has the right to refuse any kind of medical care, including palliative care. Health-care providers have to respect such a refusal. But even if the patient refuses such care, it remains available as a reasonable alternative to euthanasia. Several courts hence have argued that a patient's situation is not hopeless and prospectless if the patient herself refused a reasonable alternative (e.g. District Court Haarlem, 4 July 1994). But other courts have argued that the reasonableness of a particular alternative treatment option can only be assessed by the patient. If the patient insists on remaining fully conscious and hence refuses certain effective palliative drugs that would diminish her awareness, those drugs are not a reasonable alternative. The physician now has no alternative left but to end the patient's life.

A classic example of such a scenario was the assistance in suicide rendered by psychiatrist Dr Chabot (for the details of this case, see below). The patient had lost her husband and both her sons. Dr Chabot proposed antidepressants to relieve her grief-related depressed mood but she refused. Chabot remembers her explaining: 'Antidepressants will perhaps make me feel somewhat better, but what does it alter for me? Mourning my children means to let them go and to become a different person. That is exactly what I do not want: I don't want to become a different person from the one I was when I was a mother and happy.' According to Chabot, 'She did not want to feel better. She wanted to die ... Her refusal of antidepressants was "well-considered".'[172] Thus we find that this criterion evaporates as an objective criterion that is independent from the patient's subjective request for euthanasia. Whenever a patient explicitly requests euthanasia, which means that she does not want other forms of treatment to relieve her suffering, by definition there is no alternative left.

The patient's condition

The single most important criterion that distinguishes euthanasia from other forms of requested termination of life is the medical condition of the victim. As we have seen, the Dutch legislature from 1886 believed that *nobody* may end another person's life, even if the victim explicitly requests to be killed. Although such a request implies that the murder is no longer a violation of that individual's right to life, it is still an affront against the sanctity of human life in general. Hence, the legislature prohibited murder (Article 289) as well as homicide at the victim's request (Article 293). Most people, even staunch proponents of legalized euthanasia, still believe that homicide at the victim's request ought to remain punishable. They only want to make an exception if the person desiring death is severely ill. It is the fear of dying a prolonged death from some dreadful disease that drives the euthanasia movement. So we find that the new law of 2001 states that termination of life at the victim's request is lawful only if the victim is a patient whose suffering is prospectless and unbearable. In all other cases, the old Article 293 remains in force.

The earliest euthanasia cases adjudicated by Dutch courts all concerned patients who were either terminal or at least severely ill from somatic diseases such as cancer and advanced multiple sclerosis. But by the end of the 1980s, the nature of patients' suffering began to include psychiatric illnesses. In 1989, the District Court of Rotterdam judged a family physician who had assisted in the suicide of a psychiatric patient. The case made it all the way to the Supreme Court (28 May 1991). Although the Supreme Court pointed out that several other requirements of due care were violated (such as inadequate use of alternatives and no consultation with an independent physician), it did not protest against the fact that this patient's suffering was caused by mental as opposed to somatic illness.

Then came the famous case of psychiatrist Dr Chabot. He had ended the life of a patient who was depressed. Her suffering was severe but, according to Dr Chabot himself, her depression was related to her grieving and there were no psychotic features.

Ms B was 50 years old when she died in 1991. She had married at age 22 and although two sons were born, her marriage had been bad from the very start. Then the oldest son, with whom she had a very close, even symbiotic relationship, committed suicide. Her husband began to drink and beat both her and their surviving son. She became suicidal and it was only her care for her remaining son that kept her going. For a short while, she was hospitalized in a mental clinic and treated, but without much success. After her father died, she left her husband and in 1990 was officially divorced. Then disaster struck once more: her remaining son was diagnosed with a malignant lung tumour. He died in May 1991. The same evening that her son had died, Mrs B, planning to be buried together with her son, committed suicide. But her attempt failed. She then contacted the Dutch Society for Voluntary Euthanasia, who routed her to psychiatrist Dr Chabot. He offered therapy, aimed at detachment from her deceased family, but she refused. In September of that year Dr Chabot provided her with the necessary means to end her life, which she did.

The District Court of Assen noted that the discussion as to whether Mrs B was even mentally ill had yet to be settled. But that issue was not decisive. The Court argued that the source of suffering is irrelevant and accepted *force majeure*. On appeal, this argument was accepted by both the High Court of Leeuwarden (30 September 1993) and the Supreme Court (21 June 1994). Note that the Supreme Court rejected *force majeure* because the physician had failed to consult another physician, which the Court deemed necessary if the source of the suffering is not somatic. In view of the irreversibility of PAS, the Medical Disciplinary Court reprimanded Dr Chabot for agreeing to PAS without insisting on treatment first and his failure to have the patient examined by an independent psychiatrist.

The Chabot case represents a major shift in the debate about euthanasia. Suddenly, people who are not patients in the common sense of that term, that is, people with a diagnosed trauma or illness, could be euthanized. But there was one more limit to be pushed. Mrs B at least had a history of several major mental traumas (spousal abuse, divorce, loss of two children), resulting in hospitalization. Her depression, though not psychotic in nature, had been severe. What if a person without any such history would want to have euthanasia? A person who maybe was old and tired of living, but not suffering from any major illness or even mental trauma?

Mr Brongersma had always lived an active life, first as attorney, then as researcher at the Criminology Institute of the University of Utrecht, and finally as member of the Upper House of parliament. Although he never married and had no children, he once had a large circle of like-minded friends with whom he had frequent intellectual conversations and debates. But all of that had now fallen away. According to psychiatrist Van Ree, who spoke with Brongersma before his death, his loss of joie de vivre was caused in part by his increasing scientific isolation: 'For years, he had taken a leading role in the debates about pederasty and paedophilia. Some of his earlier debating partners passed away and the political and public opinion distanced itself ever further from his views. All of this caused him to feel increasingly isolated.'[173] In 1984 he delivered a euthanasia testament to the office of his family practitioner (which he renewed in 1993 and again in 1998). In 1991 he corresponded with Professor Drion about the latter's proposal for a suicide pill and two years later asked his new family physician for such a pill. All along, his health was generally good, particularly in view of his advancing age. In 1998, now 86 years old, he had minor incontinence and some difficulty walking. Psychiatrist Dr Noll examined him for possible depression, but found no such disorder. Two weeks later, Senator Brongersma took the lethal medications (depronal and pentobarbital) that his family practitioner had supplied him with as requested, and died.

The District Court of Haarlem consulted several experts in order to determine whether Senator Brongersma's suffering had been so severe that it was indeed unbearable and prospectless. De Beaufort, professor of medical ethics, testified that his suffering may not have been somatic or mental, but it was authentic and his desire to die autonomous. This might well have made his suffering unbearable. Expert witness and psychiatrist Reus affirmed that Brongersma suffered from the meaninglessness of his life. Precisely because the source of his suffering was neither somatic nor mental, it could not be treated and hence was prospectless. Psychiatrist Van Ree would later reach the same conclusion: Brongersma's suffering was beyond prospect, because his deceased friends could not be resurrected and society was unlikely to change its negative views about paedophilia any time soon.[174]

On 30 October 2000, three weeks before the new proposal of law was voted on in the Lower House of parliament the District Court concluded that the unbearableness of suffering, unlike its prospectlessness, is a highly subjective and personal experience that cannot be verified easily. The evidence presented to the court made it likely that the physician could have reasonably concluded that Senator Brongersma was suffering unbearably. Hence, the physician's rendering assistance in suicide had been justified and he was not liable to punishment (for the verdict on appeal, see Chapter 5, pp. 165–8)

Even if one were to agree that life itself, without any serious somatic or psychiatric illnesses, can become a source of unbearable suffering, one has to wonder how that condition can cause a conflict of duties for a *physician*. The reasoning of the court would imply that physicians have a duty to relieve *any* kind of serious suffering, even if such suffering is not at all caused by either somatic or mental illness or handicap. But if a person has no serious illness whatsoever, how could a physician ever claim that (s)he is nevertheless obligated, *precisely as a physician*, to relieve that person's suffering?

We have already seen that physicians can only invoke to *force majeure* if they are truly involved in the patient's care *qua physician*. The mere fact that the person committing euthanasia happens to be a physician does not suffice when (s)he is acting foremost as a friend or spouse. If (s)he is called in with the sole purpose to end the person's life, that does not suffice either. The physician has to be involved in the medical care of the patient and out of the apparent failure of such care, a duty can arise to end the patient's life. But in the case of Senator Brongersma, there was no failing medical care. Granted, all alternative palliative therapies had failed, but only because there was no illness requiring medical therapy in the first place. Brongersma was not psychiatrically depressed, he was merely tired of living. But that is hardly a *medical* condition requiring *medical* care. It is therefore unclear how a physician could argue that he had a professional duty to assist in this person's suicide.

Guilty but no punishment

The foregoing analysis of Dutch jurisprudence has shown that from a legal perspective, the case in favour of lawful euthanasia has been weak. Euthanasia and assistance in suicide have been clearly prohibited by the legislature from 1886. The fact that the victim was a patient, explicitly asked to be killed, and was euthanized by a physician administering drugs, should not make a difference. That law remained unchanged until 2001. Yet time and again the Dutch courts, including the Supreme Court, found that physicians who killed their patients were acting lawfully. Even if the victim was not a patient in the common sense of that term, even if the available option of palliative care had simply been refused by the patient, even if the patient had never asked to be killed, physicians were found to have acted while in a conflict of duties.

Of course, there were some cases in which the appeal to *force majeure* could not be accepted because they were too outrageous and inexcusable. The courts simply had to find against the physicians and deem them liable to punishment. How then is it possible that no Dutch physician was ever sent to jail? This brings us to the last troublesome aspect of Dutch jurisprudence.

As in most other jurisdictions, the Dutch Penal Code only defines the maximum punishment, not the minimum. It is left to the judge to determine the penalty, up to the specified maximum. We have seen that the penalties for assisting in suicide, euthanasia and nonvoluntary termination of life are respectively 3, 12 and 20 years' imprisonment.

Before the 1886 law, the penalties were even stiffer. One of the old nineteenth-century cases is a classic Romeo and Juliet tragedy about a young soldier and his fiancée. These lovers could not marry and decided to jointly commit suicide. The girl's suicide succeeded, but the young man survived. In 1859, the Provincial Military Court imposed the death penalty. (On appeal, the High Military Court reversed the verdict because the old Code Pénal did *not* prohibit assisting in suicide, as does the 1886 Code.)

Of course, history repeats itself. In 1908 a young sailor shoots his fiancée at her request. When he is about to turn the gun on himself, he begins to worry that he may not have killed her – which as it turns out he did not. Instead of committing suicide, he calls for help. The District Court of Amsterdam finds him guilty of attempted murder at the victim's request and sentences him to two years' imprisonment.

These early cases are interesting for various reasons. First, they are both non-medical cases. No early cases are known involving euthanasia proper. Only in 1952 is a Dutch court for the first time faced with a medical case. Second, in spite of the tragic circumstances of these cases and the clear and explicit requests by the victims themselves, the courts did not hesitate to impose severe punishments, including the death penalty. This is in stark contrast with the manner in which the courts came to handle euthanasia cases.

We have already seen that the District Court of Utrecht, which dealt with the very first Dutch euthanasia case, found the physician guilty and rejected the appeal to his personal conscience. More interesting for our discussion here are the reflections of the court about the seriousness of the crime. The court argued that the crime described by Article 293 is very serious indeed. In order to discourage other physicians from committing the same crime, the court deemed it necessary to impose a stiff sentence of one year imprisonment (but turned it into a probationary punishment because it was only the first case of euthanasia in the Netherlands).

When in 1973 the District Court of Leeuwarden was faced with the second euthanasia case, the stern language of the 1952 verdict had changed to a much more forgiving tone. Like the Utrecht Court, the Leeuwarden Court imposed a probationary sentence. But instead of one year, it was only one week imprisonment. The court justified this lenient sentence by pointing out that the motives of the physician 'most certainly were absolutely honourable'.

It so happened that the next two cases were not committed by physicians. In 1981, a man assisted in the suicide of his wife who had a history of psychiatric illnesses, had been hospitalized three times and feared commitment for the remainder of her life. She pressured her husband to assist in her suicide. However, both the District Court of Rotterdam and the High Court of The Hague rejected the man's appeal to *force majeure* because he could have freely decided not to assist in his wife's suicide. The District Court originally imposed a probationary sentence of one month's imprisonment; but on appeal the High Court changed it to six months' non-probationary. It pointed out that the husband had failed even to examine whether alternative and legal means of relieving suffering (e.g. expert medical interventions) could have been used. He had failed both as citizen and as spouse and had shaken the legal order.

One wonders what the High Court would have done if the husband had been a physician. In the 1973 case, the suspect had been a close family member as well (a daughter rather than a husband). In both cases, the court found that alternative and legal means had simply been neglected by the offender; in both cases an appeal to *force majeure* was rejected. Yet the Leeuwarden Court imposed a mere one week's probationary imprisonment, even though the crime of murder at the victim's request is a much more serious offence (punishable up to 12 years) than assistance in suicide (punishable up to only 3 years). Moreover, the Leeuwarden Court explicitly praised the daughter's motives whereas the Amsterdam High Court lambasted the husband. Why these differences if not because the daughter in the 1973 happened to have also been a physician?

A few months later, the District Court of Rotterdam (1 December 1981) had to decide in another case that it qualified as a 'euthanasia' case, even though it had not been committed by a physician. Again the Court concluded that a non-probationary sentence was indicated. It was only because of a psychiatric expert report suggesting that such a jail term would be too burdensome for 76-year-old Mrs Wertheim that the sentence was probationary.

Then came the famous 1983 Schoonheim case. On appeal, the High Court of Amsterdam reversed the earlier dismissal by the District Court of Alkmaar. It concluded that (a) the accused was indeed guilty of murder at the victim's request as specified in Article 293; (b) this article did apply to euthanasia cases; (c) Article 40 could not be invoked successfully because the court was not convinced that the physician had had no choice left but to end the patient's life. Then the High Court reached the unexpected conclusion that Dr Schoonheim nevertheless should not be punished because he had honestly believed himself to be acting in a just manner when he ended his patient's life and had acted with the necessary caution (17 November 1983).

Likewise in the 1984 case involving Dr Pols. The District Court of Groningen concluded that the physician was guilty of murder at the victim's request and had failed to successfully invoke any and all punishment exclusion grounds. Hence he was liable to punishment. Nevertheless, the court did not impose *any* punishment because the physician had sincerely believed that he acted justly.

Three years later, the High Court of Arnhem found a euthanizing physician liable to punishment. It did not acknowledge the physician's alleged sincerity. Instead, it recognized that the physician had been moved by the patient's suffering and imposed a probationary sentence of two months' imprisonment.

Then came the first case in which a patient was killed without a request for euthanasia. In fact, this patient had explicitly rejected the option of euthanasia. The District Court of Haarlem (4 April 1986) found the family physician guilty of murder, rejected *force majeure* and deemed him liable to punishment. But the court then concluded: 'Although the act, as proven, legally has to be qualified as murder, the Court points out that in this case any affinity with the concept of murder, as it is used in common parlour, is missing. For it has been established in the Court proceedings that the suspect has acted out of compassion and genuine concern for what he believed to be his patient's interests.' Still, the court was concerned that failure to impose a punishment, or a symbolic punishment only, might send the wrong message. The court hence imposed a probationary sentence of one week.

Two years later, the District Court of Almelo (1 March 1988) found a physician guilty of murder because he had ended a patient's life without any request from either patient or family. He had not consulted with other physicians and failed to consider and use alternative means of relieving suffering. But again the court explicitly stated that it did not question the physician's sincerity and benevolence. What distinguishes this case from previous medical murders is that this physician had ordered a nurse to inject the lethal dose. But even this fact did not seem to affect the sentence: a probationary sentence of six months' imprisonment.

On 24 October 1995 the District Court of The Hague found a family practitioner guilty of murder because he had ended his patient's life without a request from the patient. Instead, the children of the patient had asked to end her life. Moreover, there was no medical need requiring euthanasia; the guidelines from the hospital as well as the Royal Dutch Medical Association were violated; and no attempt at deliberation with colleagues was made. The court was not even fully convinced about the alleged benevolent motives of the physician and quite perturbed by the fact that the physician had ordered a significant increase of morphine (intended to cause the patient's death in a short while), but next left the hospital knowing he would only be reachable again in a week. Taking all of this into consideration, the court imposed a sentence of three months' imprisonment, probationary.

The same story goes for the District Court of Leeuwarden. On 8 April 1997 it issued its verdict against a physician who had committed euthanasia. It blamed the physician for violating the consultation require-ment and several other requirements of due care, with which the physician was well acquainted as a member of the Royal Dutch Medical Association. No *force majeure* in any form was accepted: sentence six months' impri-sonment, probationary.

We have already seen (p. 113) that on 21 February 2001 the District Court of Amsterdam imposed no punishment at all, not even a proba-tionary sentence, on Dr van Oijen. (On appeal, the High Court of Amsterdam would later impose one week's probationary imprisonment.) According to the District Court, he had acted at the request of the daughters while the patient did *not* want euthanasia. Many requirements of due care were violated. He failed to apply due medical care, using the alloferine he happened to be carrying in his bag and which had expired almost two years ago. His appeal to *force majeure* was rejected. Nevertheless, the court found that Dr van Oijen had been very much moved by the patient's plight, acted honourably and conscientiously, and in accordance with what he believed to be in the patient's best interest. It was merely a 'misjudgement' on his part, so the court concluded.

The message to Dutch physicians was clear: Given the illegality of euthanasia and murder, we have to impose a sanction; but we would rather not because we, the judges, appreciate what you are doing and do not consider it morally wrong. And the physicians understood. By 1995, only 6 per cent of physicians mentioned 'fear of legal consequences' as one of their reasons not to report euthanasia. Chabot, the psychiatrist who assisted in the suicide of a patient with no somatic illness, was found guilty by the Supreme Court in 1995 but only given a probationary sentence, would later tell an interviewer: 'The fact that the Supreme Court didn't punish me makes me feel as if I have not been convicted. ... The phrase "without punishment" makes it clear that there was no flaw in my moral reasoning and ... no major criticism of my professional conduct. Given the excep-tional circumstances of the case, no terminal phase of a physical illness, unbearable suffering from a psychic source only, this is about as far as the Supreme Court could and would possibly go in its endorsement of physician assisted suicide.'[175]

The role of the prosecutor

Until 1 April 2002, when the new law legalizing euthanasia was finally activated, physicians who ended patients' lives or assisted in their suicide were always at risk of being prosecuted and found guilty of a crime. We have seen that the threat of punishment was rather toothless. Not a single physician was ever sent to jail. As the 1980s came to an end, the courts had established a routine of dismissing cases based on *force majeure*. The most egregious of cases that were prosecuted resulted in probationary sentences only. Critics abroad concluded that euthanasia was tolerated; many even thought that euthanasia had already been legalized.

Although euthanasia was decriminalized in fact, proponents of euthanasia were quick to point out that it was not by law. Physicians were still at risk of being prosecuted. Police officers would come to the physician's office and treat him or her like any other suspect. There would be paperwork and court proceedings, and worst of all was the nerve-wrecking uncertainty as the legal proceedings moved at their typical slow pace.

The numbers in Table 4.2 show that this fear on the part of physicians was rather unfounded. In the 1980s, the number of euthanasia cases brought to the attention of the combined Dutch prosecutors skyrocketed from a handful in the beginning of that decade to more than 300 by the end. Yet the number of cases actually prosecuted did not increase at all. It never got over four cases per year and in some years no physician was prosecuted.

Still, physicians complained they did not have enough legal security. They sought complete immunity from prosecution. In 1984, a family practitioner ended the life of a terminally ill patient in the final days of her life. Not only was he so sure about his case that he did not consult another physician prior to committing euthanasia, but he also believed that his case should be immediately dismissed by the prosecutor. But the prosecutor decided otherwise and brought the case to court. The physician then asked the District Court of Almelo to dismiss the case and when (on 3 January 1986) it did not, he appealed against the verdict. On 15 October 1986 the High Court of Arnhem found *for* the physician. This time the prosecutor appealed, but to no avail. On 23 June 1987 the Supreme Court confirmed the verdict of the High Court: the physician had been correct in his expectations and should not have been prosecuted in the first place.

Euthanasia proponents had won an important victory. The Supreme Court verdict fundamentally changed the role of the prosecutor.[176] In future, prosecutors would not only think twice, but probably ten times before prosecuting a euthanizing physician. If a physician who violated a major requirement of due care had successfully fought prosecution, what point was there in prosecuting any euthanasia cases? Add to this the record number of euthanasia cases in which the judges accepted *force majeure* or imposed no sentence, and one can easily see that there was little point in prosecuting physicians. Indeed, while the number of euthanasia cases reported to the authorities continued to increase exponentially from 5 in 1982 to more than 2500 in 1998, the prosecution rate decreased from 25 per cent to 0.04 per cent.

Table 4.2 Prosecution of reported cases of euthanasia and PAS*

Year	Reported	Prosecuted
1982	5	0
1983	8	2
1984	16	3
1985	27	4
1986	84	2
1987	126	3
1988	184	2
1989	338	1
1990	486	0
1991	866	1
1992	1,201	2
1993	1,304	3
1994	1,487	3
1995	1,466	1
1996	1,689	0
1997	1,986	0
1998	2,590	1
1999*	2,216	0
2000	2,213	1
2001	2,054	0
2002	1,883	0

* As of 1999, the columns concern cases reported by physicians themselves to the authorities. In rare cases, unreported cases nevertheless become known to the authorities and are prosecuted (an example is the PAS case, Chapter 3, pp. 64–5).

Legalization of euthanasia

On 10 April 2001, a majority of the Upper House voted a new euthanasia bill into law (the complete text of which can be found in Appendix II). This was not the first time a bill to legalize euthanasia had been submitted to parliament. We have already seen in Chapter 2 (p. 52) that as early as 1984, two parliamentary members of the liberal-democratic party D66 submitted one. Pressured by this bill, the Dutch government (in which the Christian Democratic Party CDA held the lead) advanced a much more modest proposal that would not legalize euthanasia but formalize the notification procedure and the requirements of due care. Nine years later, the latter bill was accepted by parliament, while the more liberal D66 bill was rejected.

But this middle ground did not appease proponents of complete legalization. They got their chance when in the mid-1990s the CDA was finally voted out of power and a new coalition government was created that included the socialist labour party PvdA, the right-wing liberal party VVD and the aforementioned D66. In 1998, a new bill was advanced by MPs of all three parties. After minor changes, the same bill was adopted by the government and resubmitted to parliament. It is this bill that on 29 November 2000 was accepted by a majority of the Lower House and on 10 April 2001 finally made it through the Upper House of parliament.

In essence, the new law does three things. First, it revises Articles 293 and 294 of the Penal Code, legalizing euthanasia and PAS. Second, it stipulates the requirements of due care which the physician must abide by in order to be immune against punishment. Third, it delineates the process for reporting and evaluating euthanasia cases.

Legalization

In an attempt to counter criticism from abroad, the Dutch government has insisted that the new law does not legalize euthanasia. After all, paragraph 1 of Article 293 (which is the same as the old Article 293) still prohibits any and all forms of homicide at the request of the victim. And the new paragraph 2 merely provides a punishment exclusion ground for euthanasia by physicians, akin to the more generic exclusion ground included in Article 40 *(force majeure)*. Thus, a judge can always reject the appeal to paragraph 2 when the conditions specified therein are not met.

However, this line of argumentation is flawed. It is true that a physician who butchers his patient and then claims he committed euthanasia can still be prosecuted; but so can the surgeon who embarks on a dangerous operation while drunken, killing the patient in the process. It would be rather awkward to claim that surgery is still illegal in the Netherlands but surgeons who meet the requirements of due care are immune to punishment. Rather, surgery is legal, but the surgeon who butchers his patient can and will be prosecuted. The new law on euthanasia does exactly the same thing. It legalizes euthanasia, but if the requirements of due care are not met, the physician can still be prosecuted.

Indeed, under the new law physicians who commit euthanasia in accordance with the requirements of due care will never be in contact with the legal authorities. They have to submit a report to the municipal coroner and this report will be reviewed by one of the regional review committees. But if approved by the committee, the case will not be advanced to the prosecutor and no legal proceeding will ensue.

The same is true for physicians who assist in a patient's suicide. The old Article 294 prohibiting such assistance has remained in force, but physicians are excluded if they fulfil the requirements of due care. There is one interesting change, however. Physicians may not 'incite' another person to commit suicide; they may only provide means or assist in the suicide. It remains to be seen how this 'inciting' of suicide will be interpreted by the courts. After all, some proponents of euthanasia are already arguing that physicians should make euthanasia and assisted suicide a topic of discussion with their patients. If patients do not bring up the topic themselves, physicians should not shy away from doing so. Whether the courts will consider 'bringing up the topic' a form of 'inciting' remains to be seen (see Figure 4.2).

Figure 4.2   Articles 293 and 294 of the Dutch Penal Code, 2001

Article 293 Dutch Penal Code, as amended by the law of 2001

1 A person who terminates the life of another person at that other person's express and earnest request is liable to a term of imprisonment of not more than 12 years or a fine of the fifth category.
2 The offence referred to in the first paragraph shall not be punishable if it has been committed by a physician who has met the requirements of due care as referred to in Article 2 of the Termination of Life on Request and Assisted Suicide Act and who informs the municipal coroner of his actions in accordance with Article 7 second paragraph of the Burial and Cremation Act.

Article 294 Dutch Penal Code, as amended by the law of 2001

1 A person who intentionally incites another to commit suicide is liable to imprisonment of not more than three years or a fine of the fourth category, where the suicide ensues.
2 A person who intentionally assists in the suicide of another or provides him with the means thereto, is liable to imprisonment of not more than three years or a fine of the fourth category, where the suicide ensues. Article 293 second paragraph applies *mutatis mutandis*.

Requirements of due care

In addition to revising the criminal law, the new law also provides detailed guidelines for the practice of euthanasia. In fact, these guidelines are not very new. As we have seen, the various court decisions in the 1980s had already resulted in all kinds of guidelines. In 1987, a bill was proposed that reduced the punishment for requested murder to four-and-a-half years, specified that good palliative care should not be considered requested murder even if death ensued, and provided a list of requirements of due care. The law did not pass. But in 1990 the Minister of Justice issued a similar list of requirements as part of a formal notification procedure.

Since euthanasia was a crime, the authorities could not legally expect physicians to notify them of their actions. No suspect is legally required to assist in his own conviction, but without notification, it would be impossible to regulate the practice. In 1993, parliament decided in favour of a typically Dutch manoeuvre: Formally issue guidelines how to commit a crime and next expect the physician to report the crime to the authorities. The new law from 2001 incorporates these guidelines and the notification procedure from 1993.

The 2001 law states that the 'requirements of due care' which the euthanizing physician must fulfill in order to be immune from punishment are as follows. The physician:

(a) holds the conviction that the request by the patient was voluntary, well-considered and lasting
(b) holds the conviction that the patient's suffering was prospectless and unbearable
(c) has informed the patient about his situation as well as about his prognosis
(d) holds the conviction, together with the patient, that there was no reasonable alternative solution for his situation
(e) has consulted at least one other independent physician who has seen the patient and has formed an opinion about the requirements of due care listed above under (a) to (d)
(f) has terminated the patient's life with due medical care.

The question arises whether these six requirements are robust. The first one is simply part of the definition of 'homicide at the request of the victim' (see p. 112). Without a voluntary, explicit and lasting request by the patient, there is no 'express and earnest request' as specified in the first paragraph of Article 293. Thus, the first requirement of due care merely duplicates the first paragraph of Article 293.

Requirement (b) appears to be new. There has to be suffering and the suffering has to be prospectless and unbearable. But as we have already seen, even a healthy person who is not diseased or handicapped by any objective medical standard, but simply tired of living, can be suffering unbearably. Without disease, illness or handicap, the physician cannot reach an objective, scientific diagnosis. The physician will have little choice but to take the person's word that his suffering is unbearable. Thus, this second requirement of due care collapses into the first.

The third requirement specified under (c) is simply the requirement of informed consent that applies to any and all medical interventions. If, as the last requirement (f) already states, a physician has to terminate the patient's life with due medical care, informed consent is already included there. Thus, the third requirement collapses into the last.

As is true of the second requirement, the fourth requirement collapses into the first. Although the text seems to suggest that the physician has to form his or her own opinion regarding the patient's condition, the choice of words is not accidental. The text does not use the word 'and'; it states 'together with the patient'. The Explanatory Note leaves no doubt that the patient has the final say in this regard.[177] The patient can refuse any option (s)he deems unreasonable, thereby turning euthanasia into the only remaining option. Of course, the physician does not have to agree with the patient and may refuse to perform euthanasia. But the physician may also go ahead and kill the patient. Even if the physician does not agree, believing there are reasonable alternatives, (s)he can still justify euthanasia by simply pointing out that the patient had rejected all those other options.

The addition of the fifth requirement is remarkable in view of the jurisprudence. Even the Supreme Court did not think that consultation is always necessary. However, the language of this fourth criterion is very weak. It merely states that the consulted physician has to form an opinion regarding the aforementioned four requirements of due care. It does not require consensus between both physicians.

The sixth and last requirement does not entail a new demand. As pointed out earlier, it simply states that the physician must act in accordance with the standards of good medical practice, as any physician is always required to do. This includes informing the patient; it includes obtaining the patient's consent; and it often includes consultations with other colleagues when the decision at hand is very difficult.

In short, the new law does not set any new, stricter or even more precise requirements of due care for the practice of euthanasia. It does, however, create two new expansions of the already widespread practice of euthanasia. First, it specifically states that a person does not need to be competent when euthanized (Article 2, § 2). The patient can make a request for euthanasia in writing in advance of becoming incompetent, a kind of 'euthanasia testament' or 'living will for euthanasia'. The law thus inherits all the problems that living wills typically invoke. Consider, for example, a patient in the beginning stages of Alzheimer's disease. She fears a downhill slope and writes a living will requesting euthanasia. Can this patient, who has never before been demented and does not know how her brain, mind and attitudes will be affected by the disease, accurately predict that her wish for euthanasia will be lasting and the only reasonable alternative, as stipulated by requirements (b) and (d)?

Even more troublesome is the fact that minors can request euthanasia as well. The law stipulates that a minor between the ages of 16 and 18 who appears mature can be euthanized at his or her request, provided the parents have been consulted (Article 2, § 3). Note that the parents cannot stop the euthanasia. In fact, they may not be able to stop the euthanasia of their 12-year-old child either. If the parents of a child between the ages of 12 and 16 oppose euthanasia, but the physician believes that 'serious harm' can be prevented by means of euthanasia, the physician can override the parents and euthanize a 12-year-old child at its request (Article 2, § 4).

At first sight, this paragraph (Article 2, § 4) seems to follow the Civil

Code (Book 7, Article 450, § 2) which grants minors between the ages of 12 and 16 a limited right to consent. In principle, both the minor patient and the parents must consent to the medical intervention or else it cannot be provided. But the physician can override the parents' refusal in favour of the child's consent if providing treatment will keep the patient from a serious harm. The irony is that in this article 'serious harm' generally means death. For example, a paediatrician can proceed with a blood transfusion over and against the refusal of Jehovah's Witness parents but in accordance with the consent of a mature 14-year-old if the transfusion is a life-saving intervention. How killing a child can possibly prevent a more serious harm is hard to imagine.

Notification and evaluation

The third and largest part of the new law delineates the procedure for notification and, foremost, evaluation of euthanasia. Since the Burial and Cremation Act already contains guidelines specifying how a physician should notify the authorities when (s)he has committed euthanasia, the new law had only to formalize the evaluative process. The evaluation of euthanasia is completely retrospective. In fact, Article 16 specifically prohibits any member of the Regional Review Committees from providing prospective advice to physicians who are planning to euthanize one of their patients. This is somewhat remarkable since euthanasia is now legal. While it was still illegal, the authorities evidently could not evaluate and approve euthanasia prospectively. The courts could only find in hindsight that the physician had been compelled to euthanize the patient because of *force majeure*. But now that euthanasia has become legal, it is not clear why the tradition of retrospective evaluation has been continued.

As before, the attending physician is legally required to inform the coroner that the patient did not die of natural causes but as a result of either euthanasia or assisted suicide. When the coroner receives such notice and the accompanying report, these documents will be forwarded to one of the Regional Review Committees that have been formed to evaluate all reported euthanasia cases. If approved by the committee, the physician will be informed in writing, but no report will be sent to the legal authorities. Only if the committee finds that the physician has not acted properly will the public prosecutor be informed (see Chapter 3 pp. 85–7 for more details on these committees).

Why a new law?

One of the most intriguing questions is why this formal legalization of euthanasia and PAS was necessary. As we have seen, the argument that euthanizing physicians in years past had to fear legal proceedings and imprisonment is unfounded. Of the close to 20,000 cases that came to the attention of the combined prosecutors in the last decade of the twentieth century, only 20 were actually prosecuted; in other words, about one in a thousand cases. Note that the actual number of euthanasia cases is at least twice that of reported cases, reducing the chance of prosecution even further. This rate of control does not seem very high. Most other professionals who kill their fellow human beings as part of their job (such as police officers, soldiers and – in countries were the death penalty is allowed – judges or juries) are submitted to more frequent and far more rigid reviews.

For years, the primary goal of the Dutch government has been a pragmatic one: Foster self-reporting by physicians who euthanize patients in an attempt to exert control and improve the quality of care. The question is whether the new law will fulfil this goal. First of all, the incidence of self-reporting, though rising in the 1990s, at best was 50 per cent of the actual incidence of euthanasia. More problematic is that as the guidelines became more lenient and the prosecution rate continued to decrease, the self-reporting began to decrease. In 1998, only one out of 2590 euthanasia cases was prosecuted, the lowest rate ever. Yet in 1999, the self-reporting decreased to 2216. This number further decreased to 2123 in 2000. It is unlikely that this reduced self-reporting rate reflects an actual decrease in euthanasia cases, even more so since 2000 was the year in which the new euthanasia law was accepted by the Lower House of parliament, reflecting a wider public and governmental acceptance of euthanasia than ever before in Dutch history.

It has yet to be determined what has caused this decrease in reporting incidence if not a decrease in the incidence of euthanasia itself. There are two feasible explanations. One is that the adherence of euthanizing physicians to the requirements of due care has been decreasing. These physicians quickly figured that the safest route would be not to report. The new law will have no effect on that attitude since adherence to the requirements has become a decisive condition for legal immunity under the new law. Euthanizing physicians who violate one or more of the requirements of due care will continue to hide their deeds.

The second explanation is that euthanizing physicians increasingly believe that euthanasia is normal medical practice and none of the government's business. They believe it is up to them to decide whether or not euthanasia is appropriate, together with the patient but at times even without the patient's input. The fact that the new law guarantees immunity from prosecution to physicians who abide by the requirements of due care probably will not convince these physicians. There are no committees evaluating abortions; there are no committees evaluating palliative care; why then should they submit to evaluations by these euthanasia committees?

Only time will tell whether the modest goal of the new law will be realized and the incidence of self-reporting by euthanizing physicians will increase. Unfortunately, such an increase could just as well reflect an increase in the actual incidence of euthanasia now that the final barrier has been removed and euthanasia has become legal in the Netherlands.

5 | Justifying the practice of euthanasia

Introduction

Although this book as a whole can be characterized as a discussion of the morality of Dutch euthanasia, in this chapter we want to focus on the ethical analysis of the practice of euthanasia and on the arguments that are commonly provided in the Netherlands to justify the practice. We propose to proceed in three steps.

First, we discuss why exactly the practice of euthanasia is ethically problematic. What aspects of this practice demand specific ethical justification? This first step is about making the right distinctions. Ethical debates on euthanasia are often confounding and ineffective because the various participants in the debate are really talking about different things. For example, proponents of euthanasia may argue that it is wrong to let patients suffer unnecessarily, and if patients want to discontinue life-sustaining treatment they should be able to do so. Opponents may then counter that a physician should never kill patients, even if they are suffering and specifically ask to be killed. The debate between these proponents and opponents of euthanasia is unlikely to get anywhere because they are talking about different things. From an ethical perspective, there are decisive differences between withdrawing treatment that has been refused by a patient, and ending a patient's life at her request. Each can be debated and should be debated carefully, but the two should not be debated at the same time as if they are two examples of the same practice, that is, euthanasia.

Once we have defined euthanasia and laid out the ethically relevant aspects that demand specific ethical justification, we can move to the second step. We will review ethical methods of reasoning that are commonly used by proponents and opponents of euthanasia in the Netherlands and outline the differences between these methods. Again, it is important to delineate these differences for if different participants to a debate about euthanasia are using different methods, they are not really partaking in the same debate, but in two parallel debates. Thus they are unlikely to ever reach consensus.

In the third and last step we will discuss what arguments are actually used in the Netherlands to justify euthanasia. We will focus on the two main arguments: (a) patient autonomy; (b) the suffering caused by poor quality of life. We will see that the defence of euthanasia often shifts between these methodologically diverse and at times mutually exclusive arguments, invoking whichever of the two can bolster the case at hand.

The importance of distinctions

The debate about euthanasia is replete with confusing labels and confounding distinctions, even in a country like the Netherlands where euthanasia has been discussed widely and publicly for more than 30 years. Active euthanasia is distinguished from passive euthanasia, yet it is generally unclear whether the latter refers to euthanasia by neglect or mere acquiescence in the inevitable dying of the patient. All too often the withdrawal of life-sustaining treatment that has been refused by a competent patient is labelled as euthanasia when legally it is not. Conversely, we have already seen that many Dutch physicians use high doses of painkillers to end their patients' lives, yet fail to report to the authorities because they mistakenly believe their actions do not qualify as euthanasia.

These mistaken classifications have persisted even though the District Court of Leeuwarden in the second ever euthanasia case had listed several important distinctions. The court stated that the following practices are to be distinguished from euthanasia and under certain specified conditions are not illegal:

1 Administering palliative drugs, either morphine or psychoactive agents, in climbing dosages in order to relieve the suffering, even though such drugs are known to potentially shorten the patient's life.
2 Forgoing certain life-sustaining treatments such as antibiotics in the event of a life-threatening infection.

The Leeuwarden Court verdict was never appealed against. Why then has the confusion persisted? Though clear-cut at first sight, the court's classification is actually an amalgamate. The court distinguishes euthanasia on the one hand from administering palliative medications, and forgoing life-sustaining treatments on the other. Thus it treats the latter two as comparable practices (indeed, the court enumerates them in one continuous sentence). But as we shall see in this chapter, the administration of palliative medications and forgoing life-sustaining treatment ethically are two different practices (even if compassionate care for a particular dying patient may require that we do both). In turn, each differs ethically from euthanasia, though for different reasons.

The failure first to make the right distinctions can have serious consequences. These go far beyond merely confusing the ethical debate. Klijn and Nieboer, members of the first National Committee on Euthanasia installed by the Dutch government in 1985, warned against the resulting 'hypertrophy' of physicians' responsibility. For example, if there is no distinction between actively ending patients' lives by means of a lethal injection, and passively acquiescing in their impending death, every patient death, whether procured or awaited, becomes the responsibility of the physician. The concept of a natural death evaporates. Death becomes a cultural artefact, the work of human hands. People die when and because physicians decide that they may die.

Hypertrophy of physician responsibility is likewise induced if we equate PAS and euthanasia, as frequently happens in Dutch debates. This equation implies that the physician's responsibility is not any greater when she ends the patient's life herself as opposed to assisting in the patient's own suicide. Conversely, the patient's responsibility is not any greater when she takes her own life as opposed to asking for euthanasia by a physician. Thus the hypertrophy of physicians' responsibility results in an equal demise of patient autonomy. Short of taking one's life without any involvement of a physician, it is not possible really to take full responsibility for one's own death. There is always the physician who equally shares in the responsibility. At the end of life, there is no patient self-determination, only shared-determination.

The hypertrophy of responsibility is particularly troublesome in view of the process of medicalization we have described in Chapter 2. By attributing to physicians the responsibility for all that happens to sick and dying people, sickness and death become medical phenomena themselves. Society will turn to physicians to solve even the unsolvable problem of human mortality. And physicians will come to believe that it is up to them to deal with the problem, take charge, fight death, and tame it, if necessary by procuring it.

Euthanasia versus letting go

In this and the next section, we will try to explain why euthanasia is to be distinguished from 'letting go', as well as from the provision of palliative care. In order to clarify these distinctions, we will use basic notions of ethical theory.

The commission–omission distinction

We ended the former section with a warning against hypertrophy of physicians' responsibility. Physicians are trained to be in charge, to overcome disease, to fight death. When a nurse or family member or even the patient himself suggests that life-sustaining treatment should be withdrawn or withheld, many physicians have difficulty agreeing. After all, if you have the power to extend life, yet you do not use it, that is paramount to killing the patient. This kind of reasoning on the part of the physician makes ethical sense. Human beings (and physicians in particular) are charged to be beneficent, to bring about good things. Because we have the freedom and ability to do good things, we can be held responsible both for the bad things we do and for the good things we fail to do.

In technical ethical language, freely doing something (either good or evil) is called a *commission*. Because of our freedom of choice to do or not to do it, we can be held responsible for our commissions. Whenever a surgeon transplants an organ, an internist prescribes chemotherapy, or a nurse provides cardio-pulmonary resuscitation (CPR), and the patients involved suffer iatrogenic harm as a result, we can justifiably ask the care givers 'Why did you do that?' The latter then must justify their commissions.

But we can also ask health-care providers why they did not do something. We can ask the surgeon why he did not try renal dialysis first. We can ask the internist why she did not inform the patient about the serious side effects of the chemotherapy. We can ask the nurse why he did not rush to the patient's bedside, thus failing to provide CPR in a timely manner. In all these instances the caregivers may be guilty of an *omission*; their not acting may have rendered them morally blameworthy.

The active–passive distinction

Unfortunately, the distinction between commissions and omissions is often equated with the distinction between being active and passive. It is true that caregivers who omit to provide proper care do not do what they are supposed to do. In that physical sense, they are passive. But they are not passive from an ethical perspective. Their omissions constitute ethically relevant conduct on their part. Otherwise we could not hold them responsible for their failure and blame them for being negligent. However, there are also cases in which a caregiver does not do something (i.e. is physically passive), but is not negligent. He is passive both in the physical and the ethical sense. Consider, for example, the physician who does not prescribe antibiotics because he knows that the disease is of viral origin and antibiotics hence would not work. This physician does not omit necessary treatment; he is not negligent. He simply cannot do anything because he has no means to treat the patient's infection effectively.

There are also cases in which caregivers are physically active but ethically passive. They appear to be doing something, but from an ethical perspective they are not. This happens when a nurse withdraws a feeding tube that is only making a dying patient uncomfortable; or a physician pulls the plug of a ventilator when a competent patient no longer wishes to be ventilated. From an ethical perspective, these health-care providers are stopping treatment, they are no longer treating. In short, they are not treating. Granted, the caregivers in these examples will feel as if they are doing something. Indeed, to disconnect the venous line, the nurse must do certain things. He must prepare the insertion site, tie the line, slowly withdraw the needle, and bandage the wound. The physician who discontinues artificial ventilation still has to turn the knob. The undoing of our doing still entails some physical doing. Sometimes, even our never doing something involves some doing. If a physician decides not to resuscitate the patient, she has to write a do not resuscitate (DNR) order to the other physicians and nurses.

We are also tricked by our language. Instead of saying that this patient will *no longer* be fed artificially (a *negative* formulation – something does *not* happen), we often say that the physician *withdraws* the artificial nutrition (a *positive* formulation with an *active* verb). Instead of saying that a nurse does *not* resuscitate (a *negative* formulation), we often say that he *forgoes* resuscitation (a *positive* formulation within an *active* verb). And there are many more examples: we pull the plug, stop the antibiotics, discontinue the radiation therapy, refrain from surgery, disconnect the venous line, withhold life-support technology, remove the feeding tube, switch off the ventilator. It all sounds like a commission, and yet it is not.

The foregoing examples make clear why the active–passive distinction is so confusing. Our being active physically does not necessarily coincide with ethical activity. Indeed, four different scenarios can be distinguished.

1 We are physically active and hence also ethically active (commission). This is the most common scenario in which we bring about some change and hence can be asked why we did that. Most of health care falls into this category. An obvious end-of-life care example would be the nurse who resuscitates a patient.
2 We are physically passive but ethically active (omission). This happens when we do not do something that we should have done because we were obligated to do it. Negligence falls into this category. An example would be when a nurse does not rush to the patient who is suffering a cardiac arrest (a so-called 'slow code').
3 We are physically passive and ethically passive. This happens when we do not do something where we are not obligated to do something (either because we simply cannot do something; we can but we should not do it; or we can and may do it but are not required to do it). An example would

be the physician who does not prescribe antibiotics to a patient suffering from a viral disease.

4 We are physically active but ethically passive. This happens when we are undoing some activity or preventing some activity, because we should not engage in that activity (any longer). An example would be withdrawing or withholding a feeding tube that a competent patient has refused.

Given these four very different scenarios, it would be best not to use the active–passive distinction. But if the terms are used anyway, it is important to verify what they refer to: the level of physical engagement or the level of ethical engagement. For example, when people talk about 'passive euthanasia' they could mean three very different things.

1 Sometimes the word 'passive' in 'passive euthanasia' refers to the level of physical engagement only. An example would be the Dutch paediatric surgeon who failed to operate on the life-threatening duodenal stricture of newly born baby Ross (District Court of Maastricht, 19 April 1987). The physician did not treat this condition even though surgery could have solved the patient's problem effectively and was not futile on any other medical account. Therefore, he was acting ethically even though he was not acting physically, a so-called omission. His actions are properly called euthanasia because he wanted this baby (who also had Down syndrome) to die. The omission was the means of his choice to achieve this goal.

2 Sometimes 'passive' refers to the level of ethical engagement only. An example would be the physician who withdraws a ventilator from a patient because the patient has refused further ventilation. In this case, the physician must do something physically, but he is not acting in the ethical sense of the term because he is no longer obligated to act. Indeed, he is obligated not to ventilate the patient because medical treatment of any kind always requires the consent of the patient, and this patient no longer consents. However, it would be improper to label this non-action 'euthanasia' because the physician did not intend the patient to die. Even if the patient himself intended to end his own life by refusing further ventilation, the physician simply had no choice in the matter any longer. An exception may be the case of the orthopaedic surgeon who inherited several million euros after his patient died from self-imposed starvation.[178] Even so, whenever a competent patient refuses treatment, it cannot legally be administered. Dutch law is absolutely clear on this point. Not having any choice, the physician was not acting in the ethical sense of that term. Since he was not acting, he could not direct his actions, and hence he could not intend the patient's death. He merely acquiesced in the patient's refusal.

3 Sometimes 'passive' refers both to the level of physical and ethical engagement. An example would be the physician who does not operate

on a dying patient because the surgery would not improve the patient's quality of life but only extend her suffering for a few more weeks. This physician is truly 'passive', but again not engaged in 'euthanasia'. She does not forgo the operation because she wants the patient to die. She merely acquiesces in the inevitable death of the patient.

A lot of clarity would be gained if, instead of the dual 'active–passive' distinction, we use a triple 'commission–omission/negligence–acquiescence' distinction. The crucial difference between negligence and acquiescence is whether or not we are *morally called* and hence *obligated* to do something. If our non-engagement is a failure to respond to such a call, we are guilty of negligence. But if we are not called to intervene, we carry no responsibility for letting go of the patient, for allowing the natural course of events.

Medically indicated versus futile interventions

Obviously, one of the most difficult ethical tasks is to determine when we are called to treat patients and when we may or should let nature take its course. It is clear that there comes a moment when continued medical interventions harm the dying patient. But when? Physicians have always been aware of the dangers of overtreating patients, thereby doing more harm than good. In the 'Hippocratic Corpus' (the collection of works attributed to Hippocrates) we already find warnings to physicians not to overtreat patients who are overcome by their disease. The scientific and technological advances of the twentieth century have pushed the boundaries of what is medically possible far beyond the meagre means of our Greek ancestors. But the old problem of benevolent interventions that turn out to be maleficent remains as urgent as it was 2500 years ago. Medical errors remain one of the leading causes of death.

In fact, the problem has only grown worse. The regimen of effective treatments available to ancient Greek physicians was small. Moreover, virtually none of those treatments could really modify the condition of terminally ill patients. All that would be required of the ancient Greek physician is the humble admission that he was powerless in the face of death. The problem for the modern physician is not that she is powerless; the problem is that she is too powerful. Van den Berg's 1969 *Medical Power and Medical Ethics* which started the Dutch euthanasia debate was first and foremost a bitter complaint against overtreatment of patients.

In the literature one can find many labels for overtreatment. The Hippocratic documents talk about patients who are 'overmastered' by their disease, rendering the physician 'powerless'. Catholic ethicists have coined the distinction between 'ordinary' medical interventions (that may not be forgone by terminally ill patients and their care providers) and 'extraordinary' interventions (that may be forgone in the face of death). The

Vatican Declaration on Euthanasia from 1980 concedes that this distinction may not be sufficiently clear and instead proposes to use the terms 'proportionate' and 'disproportionate'. Still others have contrasted medical treatments that are 'normal', 'basic' or 'routine' from those that are 'overzealous', 'heroic' or 'experimental'. More recently, the terms 'futile' and 'futility' have come into vogue.

Dutch authors have coined the distinction between medical treatments that are *zinvol* from those that are *zinloos*.[179] There is no adequate English translation, other than 'meaningful/meaningless' or 'purposeful/purposeless'. These tentative translations reveal that the level of effectiveness is not decisive. Medical treatment that is ineffective (e.g. antibiotics for a viral infection) is obviously *zinloos*. But not every effective treatment is *zinvol*. The treatment must also have 'meaning' and 'purpose' for the patient involved. Unfortunately, the Dutch have not been able to clarify exactly when and why effective medical treatment loses its meaning and purpose. Thus, it remains as difficult for Dutch physicians as it is for English-speaking caregivers to distinguish between treatments that are medically indicated and hence must be offered to the patient (lest the physician is guilty of negligence), and those that have become *zinloos* or futile and hence may or must be forgone.

We do not pretend to solve this medical-ethical quandary in this book. However, we cannot evade the problem either, particularly in a book on euthanasia. Hence, we will stipulate a definition of 'futility', at least for the purpose of this book. We propose to define 'futile medical treatment' as treatment that cannot or is very unlikely to benefit the patient either because:

- it is ineffective (e.g. antibiotics for a viral infection)
- its effectiveness is limited to an organ or body part only and does not improve the condition of the patient overall (e.g. cardiac bypass surgery in a patient with metastatic cancer)
- it is effective but the harmful side effects of the treatment are more severe than its benefits, such that the patient overall is not benefitted (e.g. inserting a nastrogastric feeding tube in a severely demented and confused patient when this requires restraining her permanently).

The distinction between negligence and acquiescence thus hinges on whether or not the proposed medical treatment benefits the patient's medical condition overall. There is an ever greater danger in modern medicine to lose track of the patient's overall medical condition because of medicine's tendency to break the patient down into a series of separate organs, each of which is another specialist's domain.

Two further specifications must be made. First, judgements about futility are always specific to the patient involved. It is this particular patient's overall medical condition that should be improved. Cardio-pulmonary resuscitation may be medically indicated for most hospitalized patients, but not for patients with metastasized cancer because the success rate now has gone down from an average chance of 14 per cent to leave the hospital alive to less than 1 per cent.[180] But then again, a patient who really wants to be present at the impending birth of her first grandchild may consider sufficient and worthwhile even a 1 per cent probability of reversing an arrest, irrespective of a 20 per cent chance of severe neurological side effects.

Second, the fact that judgements about futility are always specific to particular patients does not mean these judgements are subjective, mere matters of opinion or the personal wishes of the patient only. A judgement of futility requires an objective assessment of the patient's condition, using scientific methods of diagnosis and prognosis, and a careful determination of the patient's medical needs, using sound methods of patient interviewing and empathic communication. The patient's own wishes are crucially important but not decisive. If a patient wants a particular medical treatment, that does not yet mean it is also medically indicated and should be administered. The reverse is true as well. If a patient does not wish a particular medical treatment, that does not yet mean it is futile.

Euthanasia versus palliative treatment

In 1973 the District Court of Leeuwarden distinguished euthanasia from forgoing futile medical treatments. We have seen that this distinction is correct indeed. The court also distinguished euthanasia from the administration of high doses of painkillers and other palliative drugs to relieve the patient's symptoms, even if those drugs are known to (potentially) shorten the patient's life. This distinction is ethically correct as well, but for very different reasons. After all, both euthanasia and palliation are commissions, interventions in the natural course of events. Hence the difference here is not between being active and being passive. The physician who commits euthanasia not only knows that the patient will die as a result of the drugs he administers but he also wants this to happen. Indeed, he wants the patient to die as soon as possible and selects drugs and dosages that will best achieve this goal. The euthanizing physician *intends* the patient's death. The palliating physician does not.

Intent (also called 'intention') is a key concept in ethics. Intent changes something from a mere natural event or unfortunate accident into chosen, goal-directed conduct for which we hence can be held responsible. In order to intend an action, it is not enough that we know about the outcomes nor even that we cause those outcomes. We must also strive for those outcomes and direct our actions accordingly. Consider, for example, the rare case of a child who dies from meningitis after a measles vaccination. The nurse who injected the vaccine knew that it could cause a lethal meningitis. She is also the one who injected the vaccine, thereby causing a perfectly healthy child to die. Nevertheless, the nurse is neither ethically responsible for the child's death nor legally liable for homicide charges because she did not direct her actions at the child's death. Hence, some ethicists would characterize this as a case of 'indirect killing'.

The same line of reasoning applies to end-of-life care. Four years after the verdict of the District Court of Leeuwarden, the following case was brought to the Medical Disciplinary Court of Amsterdam:

The patient was a 66-year-old lady who had been suffering from metastasized laryngeal carcinoma for the past two years. Radiation and surgery could not prevent near-suffocation due to laryngeal constrictions and a festering tracheal stoma. The round-the-clock need to manually clear crusts from the patient's throat caused sleep deprivation and she became ever more exhausted. The physicians offered her the option of a sedative to get some sleep and rest. They warned her that due to the sedative she might not notice becoming oxygen-deprived again and might die in her sleep. The patient discussed this information at length with the health-care team as well as family members and her minister. In the end, she decided in favour of the sedative and was given 20 mg of valium and 25 mg of phenergan intramuscularly and another 20 mg of valium intravenously. The patient fell asleep and not long afterwards died.

Four weeks later, her husband charged the hospital with improperly administering a sedative that caused his wife to die. But on 8 February 1977 the Medical Disciplinary Court decided in favour of the hospital because of the medical needs of the patient and the fact that the patient, while fully competent and upon being adequately informed about the risk of death, chose to take the sedative. The husband appealed to the Central Disciplinary Court, but it confirmed the decision of the lower court on 30 March 1978.

Consider, in contrast, the following case. It has not been published in the literature but was related to us by one of our colleagues, who is also the son in the case:

The patient was a married man, 60 years of age. Strange neurological symptoms in one hand had caused him to visit his physician. It turned out to be advanced lung cancer which had metastasized to his neck. The cancer was aggressive and soon the patient was having difficulties breathing for which he received morphine. The cancer had also metastasized to the bones causing pain. One month after the diagnosis, the patient discussed euthanasia with his family members and his family physician. Three more months of struggle followed, two more than his physicians had originally predicted even though he had decided to forgo radiotherapy. The patient was fortunate in that he could remain at home, but at the end of those four months he was exhausted. After the necessary goodbyes and in the presence of his wife and son, the family physician first injected a sedative. The relief of the induced sleep was such that the exhausted patient passed away before the subsequent lethal drugs were administered.

This case is fundamentally different from the previous one about the patient with laryngeal cancer. In the former case, the hospital physician had administered the drugs only to induce sleep. Even though he knew that the patient could subsequently die, his intent was only to induce a restful sleep. He chose his drugs and the dosages such that they would induce sleep effectively. All along, his actions were aimed at providing the exhausted patient with much needed rest and relief from her exhaustion.

The family physician in the second case also administered the sedatives to induce relief, but not relief from the patient's own symptoms. Rather, the sedative was administered to make sure that the patient would not experience the lethal muscle relaxants that were to be administered next in order to stop his breathing, a very scary experience. It was all part of a plan to induce death, except that death came sooner than expected. The difference between the two cases is further shown by the fact that the family physician in the second case, upon administering the sedatives and finding that the patient appeared to have passed away, administered a lethal dose of muscle relaxants anyway, just to be sure.

Wishing for the end versus bringing about the end

The two cases sketched in the former section clearly illustrate the difference between the intended effects of our behaviour (for which we are ethically responsible because we planned for them to happen and made sure they would happen), and so-called 'side effects' (for which we are not responsible because we could not prevent them from happening and merely tolerated them). Still, this difference is often difficult to discern when our wishes are not the same as our intentions and thus become one more confounding factor.

As pointed out, an outcome can only be qualified as intended if we direct our actions towards that outcome. It is neither enough to know that the outcome may occur, nor to wish for the outcome to occur. If we merely wish for a particular outcome but do not do anything to achieve it, it is not an intended outcome. It often happens that we wish for a patient to die soon and sigh 'if only God would come and get him!' We may be right or wrong in wishing this, but we are not responsible for his death if the patient then passes away.

The same is true for the hospital physician in the first case (p. 142). Even if he wished for the patient to die as a result of the administered sedatives, he neither selected the drugs nor adjusted the dose to bring about the patient's death. His wishes had no impact on his actions. If he wished for the patient to die, that wish remained a mere wish and never became an intention. But the family physician in the second case not only wished for the patient to die, but he also directed his actions towards that goal; the outcome of death was intended.

A caregiver can determine what is a mere wish and what is really his intent by asking: 'Would I have done something differently if I had not wished for the patient to die?' If I would have done exactly the same for another patient whom I wished to live, this patient's subsequent death was not intended (even if my actions contributed to her death). But if my medical treatment was somehow different because I wanted this patient to die, her death was intended and I am therefore (partially) responsible for her death.

The literature shows that in real life it is often very difficult for clinicians to distinguish between mere wishes and intended outcomes. One of the contributors to the book *Asking to Die* recounts how he has been involved in five straight euthanasia cases and one case where he still is not sure whether it really was a case of euthanasia. The latter case concerned a patient who required high doses of painkillers, but rejected euthanasia:

On the last day of his life, his family called me early in the morning with a great deal of urgency and said he was vomiting and in obvious pain. I went to his home at once, and administered a very high level of morphine, much more than usual, about 100 mg. He quieted down immediately, but the family made it clear that they could not hold up any longer under the strain of caring for him and requested much more social support. I organized 24-hour home care. Later that evening, they called about 9 pm with the same complaints that he was restless and appeared to be in pain. Again I went to his home, but this time gave him even more morphine than I had that morning, this time about 200 mg. I gave him the injection hoping that he would die. I returned home for a few hours, and the night shift called me to tell me he had died.[181]

Did the patient require a single dose of 200 mg to effectively relieve his pain or did this physician's wish that the patient die soon lead him to inject considerably more morphine than was needed to relieve the pain? It is not ours to judge this case. We merely point out that if he administered more morphine than was indicated to relieve the pain, he committed mercy killing. Conversely, if the patient needed the 200 mg injection to be relieved of his pain, the physician did not intentionally kill the patient.

Moved by mercy but aimed at death

A second complicating factor in the analysis of intentions are motives. These are the forces that move us to do something. Motives can be internal as when hunger, pain or fear drive us to do something; or external as when family members or poverty motivate us to act. The motives that drove someone to do what he did are likely to influence our evaluation of that person. Typically, we will be less harsh on the person who stole bread out of hunger than the person who stole the same bread merely because he hated the baker or was cheered on by fellow gang members. But in all examples the conduct remains theft, that is intentionally taking what belongs to another person.

The same is true in the area of end-of-life care. Euthanasia is commonly translated as 'mercy killing'. It is important to remember that 'mercy' may be the motive but death remains the intent. The physician who is drawn into and moved by the patient's suffering and therefore euthanizes her, still intends her to die. His goal is the patient's death and to that avail he administers the lethal drugs. When judging this physician we may conclude that he should be punished less because he was moved by pity when he killed his patient. Conversely, if another physician euthanizes her patient because she was moved to do so by pressure from the patient's family, we may not be so lenient. Nevertheless, both physicians intended their patient's death; both directed their actions towards that goal, and so both committed homicide.

Intent as ethical cover-up

We have seen that clinicians engaged in end-of-life care as well as patients and their family members often find it difficult to determine whether a particular course of action qualifies as euthanasia. Consequently, cases of intentional termination of life often end up classified incorrectly as palliative care instead of euthanasia and related forms of MPD. Some commentators have protested that it would be unfair to blame these physicians. They argue that the problem does not lie with the physicians; it lies with the distinction itself for it is not as precise as we have suggested.[182] Consider again the two cases quoted above. We have suggested that the hospital physician who administered sedatives to the lady with laryngeal cancer did not euthanize her. He knew that his patient would probably die as a result of the sedatives, but did not intend the patient to die. He only tried to offer her a much needed rest and selected the drugs and dosages accordingly. On the other hand, the family physician in the second case did intend to kill his patient. The sedatives were merely part of the overall plan to end the patient's life, as evidenced by his injecting a dose of curare-like muscle relaxants after the sedatives. But what if the family physician had not done the latter? What if he had merely given the sedatives and when those drugs unexpectedly turned out to be lethal left it at that?

We do not know the kinds of sedatives the family physician administered nor how much, but what if he administered the same drugs in the same dosages as did the hospital physician? And what if we had not been told that the administration of these sedatives was part of a plan to euthanize the patient at the latter's explicit request? In short, what if we merely knew that the family physician had administered sedatives to a terminally ill and exhausted patient who fell asleep and subsequently died? What would be the difference between this family physician and the hospital physician from the first case?

Both cared for an exhausted patient who would probably benefit from a deep sleep. Both knew that their patients were terminally ill and exhausted and might die as a result of the sedatives. Both patients fell into a much needed sleep and both died subsequently. If the conduct of the hospital physician qualifies as palliative care, why not the conduct of the family physician? Alternatively, if the conduct of the family physician qualifies as euthanasia, why not that of the hospital physician? Our critics may charge that the concept of intent does not at all clarify differences. It merely covers up whatever the ethicist wants to conceal. Whoever wants to hide the practice of euthanasia will label it all as palliative care. Conversely, whoever wants to make euthanasia practice in the Netherlands look much more widespread will call it all euthanasia.

Theoretically, this criticism is correct, but only if we can really assume that the goal of providing effective palliation and the goal of achieving euthanasia demand the exact same intervention. This assumption is seldom if ever correct. If the family physician from the second case had only administered as much sedatives as he needed to offer the patient some sleep and left it at that, we could not have qualified his conduct as euthanasia. Even if he wanted to commit euthanasia, he did not do so; he merely put the patient to sleep. Any attempt to end a patient's life effectively and expeditiously with sedatives only is sloppy, even negligent. There is far too much chance that the patient will not die as a result of the sedatives or take far too long to die. We have already seen (Chapter 3, p. 88) that in 2000 one of the Regional Review Committees found against a physician because the patient started breathing again 15 minutes after the physician had declared him dead. The physician rushed off to get advice from the local pharmacist and in the meantime the coroner arrived, only to find the patient alive.

The 1990 and 1995 empirical studies have shown that many Dutch physicians gave palliative drugs both to relieve the patient's pain and hasten death. They tried to achieve two goals with a single intervention. Good patient care often requires that several treatment goals be realized at once. We may want to keep the patient pain free but also alert and free of digestive troubles. But it does not make much sense to combine the goal of a pain-free life with the goal of death. A dead patient does not need pain-killers; conversely in order to enjoy a pain-free state one has at least to be alive.

It makes sense for a patient to say 'If you cannot keep me pain free, I would rather die.' Thus it makes sense for a physician first to keep a patient free of pain with painkillers, and only when the pain treatment begins to fail, to euthanize the patient expeditiously. But it does not make sense to render the patient pain free and then continue to increase the dose step-wise until the patient dies. If the patient is better off dead than pain free, the physician ought simply to euthanize the patient and do so expeditiously. Thus the many Dutch physicians who have administered high doses of painkillers both to relieve pain and shorten their patients' lives have pro-vided poor medical treatment doubly. First, they did not provide good palliative care because they overprescribed painkillers. Second, they did not provide good euthanasia because they used the wrong drugs to end the patient's life and consequently dragged out her dying far too long.

We conclude therefore that the concept of intent is analytically sound. As all concepts, it can be misused to cover up rather than to clarify. But if properly applied it enables a breakdown of different practices that is internally consistent and compatible with commonly held moral convic-tions. As always, the question remains as to whether the difference in intent between the physician who euthanizes his patient and the physician who causes the patient's death in the course of providing state-of-the-art pal-liative care is decisive in our moral assessment of these two kinds of con-duct. Evidently, proponents of euthanasia will not frown upon the fact that palliative care specialists at times hasten the death of their patients. But the reverse is not necessarily true. Those who believe that it is immoral knowingly to cause the death of another human being may disapprove of any physician who endangers the life of her patient, even if she does so in the course of indicated palliative treatment. Notwithstanding palliative intentions, the undeniable fact remains that the physician is the cause of the patient's death, or at least is a contributory cause to the patient's death when she continues to increase the morphine to relieve the patient's shortness of breath. Is it ever morally acceptable for a physician to risk the patient's life and, if so, when exactly?

We will return to this question in a later section, but first we need to discuss one more analytical distinction. We have covered the difference between euthanasia and forgoing life-sustaining treatment, as well as the difference between euthanasia and palliative care that unintentionally results in the patient's death. We have yet to analyse the difference between euthanasia and PAS.

Euthanasia versus PAS

One of the most striking findings from the empirical studies that has been confirmed more recently by the reports from the Regional Review Committees is the significant difference between the incidence of euthanasia and PAS. Dutch physicians have always practised euthanasia about six to ten times more often than they assist in suicide. This difference may be due in part to more patients asking for euthanasia than for assistance in suicide. An early empirical study in the mid-1980s about the Dutch practice of euthanasia and PAS suggested that requests for euthanasia are about three times more common.[183] But the same study also showed that about 75 per cent of all euthanasia requests were honoured versus only 25 per cent of the requests for assistance in suicide. Indeed, when the survey asked about their attitude towards both practices, many more Dutch physicians appeared willing to grant a request for euthanasia (79.2 per cent) than a request for assistance in suicide (20.8 per cent). This is remarkable because euthanasia is a much more serious offence than assistance in suicide, punishable with 12 and 3 years' imprisonment respectively. Most foreign jurisdictions likewise treat euthanasia and assisting in suicide differently. Oregon, the only US state that has specifically legalized PAS, still does not allow euthanasia.

While acknowledging the legal distinction between euthanasia and assisted suicide, the Royal Dutch Medical Association has claimed that there is no significant moral difference between the two.[184] Given the more prevalent rejection of PAS among Dutch physicians, the association therefore favoured the term 'euthanasia' to cover both practices. Yet in the same report, the association also expressed a preference that patients assume more responsibility for their own deaths by taking the lethal medications themselves rather than expecting physicians to administer them. But this is exactly what distinguishes assistance in suicide from euthanasia.

In the case of euthanasia, the physician (nurse, or anybody else) euthanizes the patient. The patient is the 'victim' who is being killed. The situation is less clear in PAS. This abbreviation is commonly understood to mean 'physician assisted suicide'. But that would suggest there is a patient who commits suicide, therein assisted by a physician. The 'assisted by a physician' would then specify the particular manner in which the patient commits suicide. Some patients commit suicide in secret; some commit suicide in dramatic fashion by setting themselves on fire; and some commit suicide with the help of a physician. In all cases, it is the patient who acts.

Whereas the physician commits euthanasia, it is the patient who commits PAS.

In PAS, the one who is guilty of homicide is the patient. The patient takes his own life; the physician merely renders assistance. The adverb 'merely' does not imply that PAS is simple and facile, whereas euthanasia is demanding and difficult. Rather, the term signifies that the primary and ultimate responsibility for the patient's death is borne by the patient herself. The physician may instruct the patient, write a prescription, or even prepare and provide the lethal drugs, but it is the patient who requests those drugs, accepts them, and takes them. It is this difference in responsibility that explains the difference in punishment between assisting in suicide (3 years' imprisonment) and euthanasia (12 years').

Even if the legal difference between committing euthanasia and assisting in suicide is insightful and reasonable, there certainly can be clinical scenarios in which it is difficult to determine whether the physician only assisted in the patient's own suicide, or actually euthanized his patient. There is a rather obvious difference between writing a prescription for a lethal dose of drugs which the patient then buys and consumes herself, and the injection of the same lethal dose. It is less clear what the difference is between preparing a lethal dose of medicine and handing that dose to the bedridden patient who consumes it, or injecting the same dose. It is really unclear what the difference is between placing the aforementioned lethal potion at the lips of the quadriplegic patient who cannot move any limbs, or injecting the same dose.

The suicidal patient in the first comparison has to do a lot of things in order to bring about her own death. She has to go with the prescription to the pharmacist, take the drugs home, prepare them according to the instructions, make sure she will not be found, and then consume them all. Having to do a lot also offers many opportunities to abandon the suicide attempt. So we conclude that in this case the patient is really in control. On the other hand, the quadriplegic patient who cannot move her arms, and hence cannot even bring the cup to her mouth, cannot exert any physical control over the situation. But emotionally and intellectually, the quadriplegic patient may be more in control. Provided that the attending physician would only grant the patient's request after months of deliberation, and in the course of preparing for the final injection repeatedly validates the patient's continued willingness to die, this patient may be more in control than the suicidal patient from the first comparison who may be compelled by total isolation and desperation, and one day just gets the prescription, buys the drugs, and swallows them – all within a single hour. Why, may we wonder, does the physician, who prescribes the lethal drugs simply because he is asked to do so by this desperate and lost patient, commit a lesser crime than the physician who, after managing to stall a quadriplegic patient for months, finally grants her request and injects a lethal dose? Surely both physicians intended the patient's death and both directed their actions towards that effect. Both exerted control and, most importantly, both could have refused to participate.

These examples show that there are grey areas between euthanasia and physician assistance in suicide. Hence, anybody who wishes to argue in favour of PAS only but against euthanasia may have difficulty defending that position convincingly. These grey areas may also pose difficulties for legal authorities charged with the enforcement of the laws on these two practices. Uncertain as to which of the two is the most appropriate charge, they may have to settle for a lesser charge. But such evidentiary difficulties do not undermine the validity of the distinction itself.

Referral as a form of PAS

As mentioned, it may not be easy consistently to argue in favour of PAS but against euthanasia because in both practices the physician intends the patient's death and directs his actions accordingly. For the same reason, it is only consistent for a physician who opposes euthanasia also to refuse assistance in the patient's suicide. In fact, this physician cannot even direct a patient to another physician who may be more willing to assist in that patient's suicide.

Most Dutch proponents of PAS and euthanasia concede that physicians are never obligated to grant a patient's request for euthanasia or PAS. But it is less clear whether proponents of euthanasia would also respect a refusal to refer the patient. In its 1984 *Statement on Euthanasia*, the Royal Dutch Medical Association argued that a physician opposed to euthanasia 'as early as possible must offer the patient an opportunity to contact a colleague'. A similar sentence can be found in the 1991 *Proposal for a Euthanasia Protocol* from the Dutch Society for Voluntary Euthanasia. The physician who is principally opposed to euthanasia 'must point out to the patient or his proxies that they can contact another physician who does not have such principal objections'.[185] Although the new law legalizing PAS and euthanasia that went into effect on 1 April 2002 does not stipulate an obligation on the part of the physician to refer, during the parliamentary debates the ministers of justice and health care made it clear that physicians who are principally opposed to the practice of euthanasia or unwilling to grant a request for assistance in suicide must nevertheless refer or actively help a patient find a physician who will.[186] These statements prove that, as far as these two ministers were concerned, Dutch physicians have a duty to assist in the patient's own suicide or assist in the provision of euthanasia. This assistance may be limited to a referral, but it is a form of assistance nonetheless.

Voluntary versus nonvoluntary MPD

One of the atypical characteristics of the Dutch debate on euthanasia is that the patient's request is part of the definition of euthanasia. Euthanasia is defined as ending the patient's life at his or her explicit and persistent request. This definition coincides with the text of the Dutch Penal Code. The Code does not use the term 'euthanasia' itself, but prohibits ending the life of another person at his or her explicit and persistent request. Consequently, whenever the patient has not asked for her life to be ended, and the physician does so anyway, this would not be euthanasia in the Netherlands. Instead, it is called nonvoluntary termination of life.

However, Dutch authors are themselves not consistent in the use of the term 'euthanasia'. In its reports on euthanasia from 1973 and 1975 the Health Council has used the term 'nonvoluntary euthanasia'.[187] So did the Royal Dutch Medical Association in its 1984 Statement on Euthanasia.[188] But if euthanasia means 'voluntary termination of life', the concept of 'nonvoluntary euthanasia' is a contradictory phrase. It would not be possible either to speak about 'euthanasia of newborns'[189] or 'euthanasia of minors'[190] since by definition neither newborns nor minors can voice an explicit request for euthanasia. Even the use of the term 'voluntary euthanasia' as in the name Dutch Society for Voluntary Euthanasia is problematic because it suggests that there is voluntary and nonvoluntary euthanasia.

The insistence by Dutch advocates of euthanasia on the voluntariness of euthanasia is not merely a matter of definitions; it is part of the strategy to justify euthanasia. However, Dutch criminal law does not attach the same significance to the patient's request as advocates of euthanasia do. The addition 'at the victim's explicit and persistent request' in Article 293 of the Penal Code does not signify that euthanasia differs fundamentally from nonvoluntary termination of life: that is, manslaughter. Rather, both are instances of homicide. The request merely mitigates the crime and the punishment hence is less.[191]

In April 2002, the new euthanasia law took effect which adds one more mitigating factor to the Penal Code. If it is a physician who ends the life of another person at his or her request, the physician will not be punished. If it is a physician who assists in the suicide of another person or provides the latter with the means to do so, he will not be punished either. All other people who commit the same crime remain punishable.

It is possible that this new law will result in a new Dutch definition of euthanasia in which the words 'by a physician' are added: 'Euthanasia is the act of ending the life of another person by a physician at the former's explicit and voluntary request.' Such narrowing of the definition of euthanasia is fine if it increases the clarity of the debate. However, it does not settle the crucial ethical question. The question remains as to whether and why the mere fact that a *physician* kills another person justifies the homicide. The question remains whether and why it is morally wrong and illegal for a nurse or spouse to do the same.

Likewise, the ethical question remains whether the fact that a patient asks to be killed changes the act from an evil deed into a good deed. The question remains whether it is always wrong to end a patient's life if the patient did not ask for it. We now know that Fenigsen was right when he charged in 1989 that many patients in the Netherlands are killed without their so requesting. The fact that the Dutch do not call this 'euthanasia' does not settle the ethical question whether the physicians who killed these patients were right or wrong.

Different methods of ethical reasoning

As we have seen in Chapter 2, in its earliest phase medical-ethical thinking was primarily deontological in nature. Deontology or duty-based ethics assumes that certain actions are morally wrong and should not be done regardless of the consequences. Conversely, other actions are morally right and must be done even if the consequences are undesirable. An example is truth telling. A deontologist will argue that a doctor must always tell the truth to her patients and may not lie, even if the patient is subsequently depressed by the bad news or decides on the basis of the information provided to forgo the proposed life-extending treatment. It would be wrong for the doctor to lie to her patient even if she could thereby save the patient's life.

There are various deontological theories depending on the source of these duties. Examples are revealed catalogues of duties such as the Ten Commandments that figure in the Judaic, Christian and Muslim religions. Authoritative catalogues of human rights are found in international treaties signed under the auspices of the United Nations and other international leagues of nations. Still others have tried to provide a strictly logical foundation of universally binding duties. The classic example is the German philosopher Immanuel Kant (1724–1804). He argued that one must always tell the truth because if people were allowed to lie, nobody would ever assume any more that people told the truth. Then there is no point in lying either because lying is only effective if the other person assumes one is telling the truth. Or to apply the same reasoning to the medical context: If physicians were allowed to lie to dying patients and told them they were doing just fine and still had a long time to live, patients would simply not believe physicians any more. Indeed, they could never be sure that the physician is telling the truth; after all, physicians are not required always to tell the truth.

In Chapter 2, we have already seen that up to the middle of the twentieth century medical ethics consisted largely of a series of physician duties that were absolutely binding, first and foremost the duty to protect human life. Many opponents of euthanasia, particularly those who argue from a religious perspective, still insist that human life is a sacred good that may never be taken. For example, the Dutch Roman Catholic bishops have repeatedly insisted on this point: 'It is our opinion that when a patient is not in the terminal phase of an illness, a doctor must always choose to preserve life and that in the terminal phase he/she may never actively and directly terminate life.'[192]

Deontological ethical reasoning conflicts with consequentialist reasoning. Consequentialism is the ethical theory that gives primacy to the consequences or outcomes of human conduct. According to a consequentialist, the morally right course of action (versus the wrong one) can only be determined by looking at the outcomes of each alternative course of action. Whichever of these courses yields the best outcomes overall is the morally superior course of action. Again, there are various versions of consequentialism, depending on the criteria used to assess and weigh the outcomes. Consequentialist reasoning is commonly applied in discussions about the ever-expanding cost of health care, the issue of access to care, and the allocation of scarce medical resources such as donor organs.

It is also applied in clinical-ethical discussions about the right course of action in any given case. For example, most proponents of euthanasia grant that death is itself not a good outcome. When patients ask for PAS or euthanasia, physicians should always attempt to relieve their suffering with other means first. However, the time may come when death overall is a better outcome than life. When Dr Chabot, who assisted in the suicide of his patient Mrs B, was asked about his attitude towards Mrs B's suicide, he replied: 'I did not agree with Mrs B's decision to kill herself, but I felt that the greater evil would be her dying alone.'[193] This consequentialist justification of PAS is actually quite common. Van Wijmen found that almost 40 per cent of physicians justify PAS as a way to prevent suicide.[194] If death is going to come anyway, the physician may as well assist the patient by prescribing the right kind of drugs. Or better still the physician should euthanize the patient – thus preventing the patient from taking the drugs, vomiting and emitting them.

One of the problems of this kind of consequentialist reasoning is the issue of responsibility. Consider the many patients who have died after physicians have increased the morphine dose far beyond what was needed for the relief of pain and with the explicit intent to shorten the patients' lives. Even if most of these patients probably did not die as a direct result of the morphine, even if the patients' deaths were not the result of the physicians' actions but the patients' illnesses, surely these physicians carried ethical responsibility for what they did? The fact that they intended their patients to die and acted accordingly is ethically relevant, even if they did not succeed.

In order to account for the relevance of intentions in our ethical analysis we must turn to a different method of ethical reasoning, that is, teleological reasoning. Teleology or goal-based ethics can be traced back to the Greek philosopher Aristotle (384–322 BC). This ethical theory is based on the assumption that it may not ever be possible to determine for any specific course of action in a particular situation whether it is truly good, or at least preferable to any of the alternative options. However, it is possible to determine what goals are worth striving for. Thus the primary question is what we are intending to do and, hence, what kinds of human beings we are trying to become. Again, a variety of answers can be given to this question. Whereas Aristotle sought to find the answer primarily in nature, Christian theologians would later add a spiritual dimension. Created in the image of God and uniquely ensouled, human beings must strive to realize this divine challenge in the course of their lives. In the twentieth century, the idea emerged that human beings should strive to be what they want to be, regardless of what it is they want to be.

The impact of teleological reflections on the ethical analysis of euthanasia is most visible in the debates about the goals of medicine. In Chapter 2, we have seen that the Dutch euthanasia debate was ushered in by Van den Berg's critique of the overtreatment of patients. The increasing medicalization of human dying and death in the course of the twentieth century fostered support for legalized euthanasia and PAS. The Royal Dutch Medical Association has argued that euthanasia and PAS are properly considered medical interventions. They are consistent with the goals of medicine. In opposition, the Dutch Physicians League has insisted that physicians may never engage in euthanasia or assist in a patient's suicide precisely because they are physicians. Maybe non-physicians can do so morally under certain circumstances, but the physician must always strive to be a healer. If death becomes the objective of medical treatment, the very foundation of the profession of medicine is undermined.[195]

Many conflicts in the debate about euthanasia arise because the participants approach the issue of euthanasia from a different methodological perspective. These conflicts are difficult to resolve precisely because they are fundamental. When two deontologists disagree about the ranking of the duty to extend life versus the duty to improve the quality of life, at least they both agree that duties are decisive in the ethical argumentation. But if a deontologist argues that physicians must always protect life because it is a sacred good, whereas a consequentialist argues that physicians must assist in patients' suicides in order to prevent them from dying alone, the likelihood of reaching agreement is significantly diminished, because the two speakers do not even agree as to what counts as a valid argument.

The Model of Double Effect

It is difficult to merge these different methods of reasoning into a single ethical theory and decision-making model because they each focus on a different aspect of human conduct, often at the exclusion of other aspects. Yet our moral experiences reveal that there is truth in all three approaches. Reality is richer than these different theories can capture. All of these aspects should be considered in the ethical evaluation of human conduct.

One attempt at a merger that appears to do justice to the reality of clinical care is the so-called 'Model of Double Effect'. This model was initially developed by Catholic theologians. Although it never became an official part of Catholic moral doctrine, it gained significant influence in both Catholic and non-Catholic bioethical thinking. The model borrows considerations from deontological ethics, teleology and consequentialism. The model is based on the observation that almost everything we do does not just have the desired good effects, but also unintended evil effects. Notably in the world of health care it is virtually impossible to benefit the patient without at the same time causing some harm to the same patient (and sometimes to others as well). Each medication has side effects; each surgical intervention carries some risk; even informing a patient honestly about her terminal illness may cause her to slide into depression. What is more, competent health-care providers know these side effects. But how can it be morally justified knowingly to inflict harm on one's patients?

We saw that the law has great difficulties in dealing with the problem of knowingly causing harm. Ethicists will argue that those harmful effects are known but not necessarily intended. Lawyers will counter that if a physician knows that high doses of morphine are going to suppress the breathing centre and therefore quite likely to kill the patient, but administers them anyway, surely he must have willed the patient's death or else he would not have given the drugs. The lawyer will grant that the physician was also trying to alleviate the patient's dyspnea, but the end does not justify the means. Indeed, it does not. The ethical significance of intentions is not absolute. A physician may not attempt to sustain the life of a terminally ill patient with means that severely aggravate the patient's suffering. Even if his actions are well intended, the goal of extending the patient's life does not justify any means to effectuate that goal. So we find that caring for the dying – caring for patients more generally – is often 'a mission impossible'. Interventions to relieve pain and suffering also endanger the patient's life; yet sustaining the patient's life demands interventions that are unacceptable from a palliative perspective.

In order to create some 'moral space' in which to act, the Model of Double Effect has been developed. The model assumes that people may perform well-intended interventions in spite of foreseeable evil consequences, if all of the following four conditions are fulfilled.

1 *The intervention may not be intrinsically bad.* This first condition is deontological in nature. It acknowledges that certain behaviours are always wrong, regardless of the best of intentions and the best of outcomes. But almost everything physicians and other health-care providers do is just, right and fair at least in some circumstance, even if it is a rare one. After all, medicine is about healing patients, about fostering their well-being, relieving suffering, improving their lot. It is fair to say then that most actions in the area of health care will meet the first of these four conditions.

2 *The actor may only intend the good effect(s), not the evil one(s).* This second condition is probably the most important of the four. It is the one that actually creates the 'moral space' that physicians need to practise medicine. For it specifies that if the physician knows about the bad effects, but does not direct his interventions towards these bad effects, he may go ahead and treat. That is not to say that his good intentions turn the bad effects into good effects; the bad effects obviously remain bad. But the physician is no longer morally responsible for the bad effects (provided that conditions three and four are fulfilled as well).

3 *The bad effects are not the means to the good effects.* The third condition makes sense in light of the second (but is also the condition that causes the model to be contested). The third condition in essence holds that the bad effects must be indirect effects. They may be either side effects that occur parallel to the good effects, or secondary effects that follow from the good effects. But the good effects may not follow from the bad effects. Why? If someone brings about the bad effect in order to indirectly achieve the good effect, that is, if the bad effect is the means to the good effect, the actor cannot claim that he did not intend the bad effect. For he directed his actions straight at the bad effect, and hence intended the bad effect. Granted, he did so in hopes of realizing the good effect indirectly, but that indirectly intended good outcome does not diminish the fact that he also intended the bad outcome.

It is the third condition that renders it morally licit to increase the dosage of morphine for a terminally ill patient who is severely suffering from pain and dyspnea, even though that treatment is quite likely to shorten the patient's life. But it renders euthanasia immoral even if the ultimate goal is to end her suffering. In the former example, the patient's death occurs as an unintended side effect (or indirect effect) of the morphine. In the latter case, the injection of drugs is not directed at the patient's pain relief, but at her death – with relief of suffering being the indirect consequence of her death.

4 *There must be grave reasons for allowing the bad effects to occur.* The fourth condition further narrows the 'moral space' created by the second condition. As mentioned, the bad effects remain bad. Hence they may not be disregarded. The actor must have grave reasons to knowingly cause

them. This means, first and obviously, that there may not be a better alternative treatment available that achieves the same good effects but with fewer bad effects or less bad effects. Second, the good effects achieved must be proportionate to or outweigh the harm done by the bad effects. In other words, the proposed intervention must pass the kind of calculus that is characteristic of consequentialist reasoning.

The Model of Double Effect does not specify the principle by which the good and bad effects must be compared and weighed. The physician generally will compare and balance the beneficial and harmful effects of a proposed intervention in the light of the patient's own overall interests, that is, the patient's health. Unfortunately, it is not always evident which alternative best fosters the patient's health. For example, in the area of end-of-life care, the debate continues between those who argue that human life is of the utmost value, a value that outweighs each and every other value; those who admit to the sanctity of life but do not consider life an absolute value; and those who do not consider human life a value in and of itself, but only the life that the person living it has freely chosen. The first will expect physicians to use all available means to extend the patient's life and will prohibit the use of any palliative means that endangers the patient's life. The second will expect physicians to extend the patient's life, but only if the treatments used do not add to the patient's suffering. Conversely, if the suffering becomes unbearable for the patient, physicians may relieve such suffering even though those palliative drugs inevitably endanger the patient's life. The third will allow physicians to use all palliative measures as well as end the patient's life if the latter so chooses.

The extreme positions – the first and the third in the former paragraph – are the easiest to defend. But extreme positions often do the least justice to the complexities of human life. We have seen that in the second half of the twentieth century the absolutist interpretation of the duty to extend life, coupled with a rapid increase in life-sustaining technologies, resulted in overtreatment of many dying patients without ever involving them in the decision-making process. In response to this medical paternalism, decision-making power was shifted away from the physicians to the patients. Respect for patient self-determination became the leading ethical principle, even if it meant ending the patient's life at her request. Yet neither alternative appears to do justice to the actual condition of the patient, to the experience of the patient, the reality of the life she is living. Both alternatives focus on death instead.

But before we reach this conclusion about the Dutch practice of euthanasia, we must examine in greater detail the arguments that are most commonly advanced to justify the practice. We begin with the principle of respect for patient autonomy because it has been the primary justification for the new law that legalized euthanasia and PAS. However, we will show that the reality of Dutch euthanasia practice is more paternalistic than the political debates would suggest. Instead of patient autonomy, judgements about patients' quality of life are generally decisive.

Patient autonomy

Van den Berg ended his 1969 critique of the rise of medical power with a plea for more respect for the patient in the decision-making process. Ever since, the emphasis on patient self-determination has figured prominently in the Dutch debate about end-of-life medical care. A patient may not be forced to undergo treatment, even if it is life-sustaining medical treatment. When a patient refuses such treatment, legally it must be withdrawn. Euthanasia is likewise justified with an appeal to autonomy. In fact, euthanasia is defined in terms of patient autonomy. If the patient does not request MPD, it no longer qualifies as euthanasia. There is no such thing as 'nonvoluntary euthanasia' in the Netherlands. A new term has been coined to cover such cases: 'nonvoluntary termination of life'. Euthanasia is justified precisely because the patient has voiced a persistent and voluntary request: 'The essence of justified euthanasia or PAS is the explicit request from the patient thereto', or so the *Explanatory Note* to the new law from 2002 states.[196] If a patient freely chooses death, it is only a token of respect for the patient if her physician grants the request.

But is the Dutch practice of euthanasia in accordance with this ideal of patient self-determination? Is each patient request for euthanasia or assistance in suicide truly free and never the result of any kind of coercion? Foreign critics have frequently charged that some patients are euthanized for economic reasons. Shortages of hospital beds and the rising cost of health care in general would be major motives. However, the empirical studies do not support this thesis. Whereas in 1990 one physician (out of 97 interviewed) admitted that economic factors motivated his ending a patient's life without the patient's request, in 1995 no physician affirmed that motive. Indeed, as we have seen in Chapter 2, the Dutch health-care system, though under pressure as similar systems elsewhere, still covers all Dutch citizens such that expenses arising from genuine medical needs are all covered. Unlike the United States, virtually all Dutch people have the benefit of insurance coverage for health care. But that is not to say that patients are under no pressure. Even if we disregard the despair that may arise from inadequate relief of symptoms and the certainty of impending death, there are still other subtle sources of coercion. Consider the initiation of the request for euthanasia. Any physician, whether willing to commit euthanasia or opposed to it on principle, must always take the patient's euthanasia request seriously and discuss it with the patient. After all, such a request reveals that the patient is fearful of the future, becoming desperate, or is suffering from unrelieved pain and other symptoms. These kinds of issues must always be addressed conscientiously if we want to make headway with palliative end-of-life care. Thus physicians must respond to a request for euthanasia or PAS. But it does not follow that physicians must also initiate this process by asking the patient whether she has thought about euthanasia, is contemplating euthanasia, or has written a euthanasia testament, let alone suggest that she may want to consider euthanasia and write a testament. Although patients who had been thinking about euthanasia but dared not raise the issue may feel relieved that their physician broached the topic, patients who would not want euthanasia yet are desperate or fearful may sense that they ought to consider euthanasia. At the very least, they will know that their physician considers euthanasia a valid option, a proper course of medical treatment. The physician may immediately follow with the assurance that euthanasia is an option only if the patient wants it herself, but the seed of doubt has been sown.

This seed may begin to grow if fertilized by other subtle messages that confirm the validity of the euthanasia option. Family members would be the primary sources of such messages. The first empirical study by Van Wijmen already revealed that almost 40 per cent of physicians surveyed in 1985 considered 'unnecessary suffering of the immediate surroundings' a justification to commit euthanasia or PAS.[197] We do not know whether this consideration actually motivated the practice of euthanasia and, if so, to a significant degree. It will be difficult empirically to assess the presence and impact of such family pressure. The fact that physicians granting the 3600 requests of euthanasia/PAS in 1995 believed that 98 per cent of the time the request was fully the patient's own does not prove there was no pressure from the family. Maybe we can conclude that the physicians involved did not notice pressure from family members. But there is also the possibility that they did not admit, anonymity notwithstanding, that they granted a request for euthanasia knowing that the patient was pressured by family members. Indeed, in two of the three annual reports of the Regional Evaluation Committees now available, the committees expressed their concern about family pressures.[198] In one instance in 2000, the committee concluded that because of such family pressure – that is, giving in to the pressure – the physician did not meet the requirements of due care.

Indeed, we do know that there is family pressure. For such pressure was listed by the physicians surveyed in 1990 and 1995 as one of the reasons *not* to grant the patient's request for euthanasia or PAS. In 1995, pressure from family members and the resultant reduction in freedom of choice on the part of the patient was a reason to refuse in 10 per cent of the 2000 refused requests (up from 4 per cent in 1990).[199]

Second, we know that 17 per cent of patients whose request for MPD was granted in 2001 (up from 13 per cent in 1995) stated they did not want to be a burden on their family members any longer. Data on nonvoluntary termination of life reveal that in 1995 approximately 900 patients were killed without their issuing an explicit request for euthanasia.[200] The physicians involved admitted that in 38 per cent of cases this was done (among others) because the family could no longer bear the burden.

It may be difficult for a family practitioner who only sees his or her patient intermittently to spot the presence of subtle pressure exerted by family members. It is even more difficult to determine the pressure exerted by the larger socio-cultural context. Education, popular and mass media, and the entertainment industry all emphasize by word and image the importance of health, fitness, youth, enjoyment, independence. These are the goals worth striving for. Conversely, handicaps, old age and dependence all render life less worth living. Patients are also impacted by these repeated messages. When euthanasia is presented as a way for patients to regain control over their lives and to manage their own mortality – and we have already seen that it frequently is (see Chapter 2) – many patients may be persuaded that the option of a self-chosen death is preferable to submission to disease and the care of others.

This idea of a human being as *causa sui*, producing his or her individual well-being, always remaining in control of his or her life and existence, is not new. In the fifth century AD, Pelagius argued that human beings possess sufficient powers themselves to achieve their own perfection. And since perfection is possible, it is also obligatory. His contemporary Augustine criticized and relativized these perfectionist ideals as a denial of human frailty and a refusal to accept that human life in principle is uncontrollable and beyond personal autonomy. Nevertheless, this ideal of human perfection through independence and self-determination has retained its appeal, as modern debates about and practice of euthanasia reveal.

It is perhaps most evident in the drive towards euthanasia testaments. Prior to the new law, patients' requests for euthanasia or PAS could only be granted if they were verbalized by a competent patient. But the new law has made it possible for any competent person to write a kind of living will declaring that he wants euthanasia if certain conditions (e.g. advanced dementia) become reality. As is true of other living wills, this euthanasia testament only becomes operative when the patient has lost his competence to make decisions about his own care. Once the conditions stated in the testament become reality (e.g. the patient's dementia has advanced), the physician may euthanize the patient based on the testament, even if at that time the patient no longer knows what euthanasia is, let alone can confirm the request. It is even possible on the basis of such a testament to euthanize a patient who is no longer suffering from pain or other symptoms (e.g. when the patient has slid into a persistent vegetative state). Prior to the new law, in such cases euthanasia was not possible because the criterion of unbearable suffering was not (or no longer) met.

The legal acceptance of these euthanasia testaments underscores the

Pelagianistic tendencies in the euthanasia debate. People may (and should?) take charge of their own lives and manage their own mortality. In this manner, all physical demise, suffering and dependence on others can be prevented altogether. A most telling example is the model testament proposed by the Dutch Society for Voluntary Euthanasia. It advises patients who do not want to be admitted to a nursing clinic to specify in their testament that they refuse such admission if it would become necessary because of the dependence on extensive or advanced care from others, and request euthanasia instead.[201]

Unbearable suffering and the patient's quality of life

At first sight euthanasia testaments appear to be the ultimate operationalization of patient autonomy. They enable a patient to retain control over his or her life even into the phase of incompetence. But this sense of control is largely illusionary. Euthanasia testaments are problematic for the same reasons as are living wills more generally.[202]

First, patient choices are genuinely free only if they have been fully informed. In a normal informed consent procedure, the doctor informs the patient of the diagnosis, several treatment options, the prognosis with and without each of those options, and all of their side effects. The patient has the chance to ask additional questions and only if she understands her predicament adequately is the subsequent patient consent valid. But this process of information is very different in the case of a living will. People are expected to write these wills before they fall seriously ill. There may not be a specific diagnosis and hence no clarity about the treatment options and little information about the prognosis. The patient must guess what illness will overcome her, what treatment options will be available at that later time, and how effective they will then be. The physician cannot be of much help either because he is no better than the patient at predicting the future.

Second, the patient must predict how she will feel when any of the illnesses listed in the living will overcome her. But it is difficult to predict one's own feelings, particularly if one has never experienced the condition. Consider the example of dementia. This disease is dreaded by many because of its devastating impact on the mind. When dementia advances, not only does the patient forget who we are, but she no longer appears the same person to us. The foresight of changing into somebody we are not, into an unknown person, frightens us. But the very same fact also makes it impossible to truly predict what life will be like should we fall prey to dementia. Our prediction that we will prefer death over living on with dementia is a mere guess, not an informed decision.

Because the future by definition is unpredictable and holds an unlimited number of possibilities, a living will must always be written in a generic manner so that it captures many of those possibilities. For example, instead of writing that she does not wish to be resuscitated if she ever suffers from metastatic cancer, the patient may write that she does not wish to undergo life-sustaining medical interventions if she has become terminally ill. Or even more generally, she may write that she does not want any life-extending medical interventions once her suffering has become unbearable, preferring euthanasia instead.

But now the third problem becomes visible. The euthanasia testament has yet to be interpreted by the patient's caregivers. The patient herself has become incompetent to make decisions about her own health care so she cannot do the interpreting. Instead, the caregivers must do it for her. They must assess whether the dementia is indeed advanced, whether the patient has become terminally ill, whether the suffering has become unbearable. But can they do so? The caregivers may be able to determine whether there are still prospects for improvement via medical treatment and other care interventions. But only the patient can determine whether her suffering is unbearable. This is exactly what distinguishes the criterion of prospectless suffering from unbearable suffering. It is up to the patient and only the patient to determine whether his or her suffering is still bearable. In the words of family physician Wibaut, 'the reason as to why a patient believes that his suffering has become unbearable is nobody else's business'.[203]

We thus find the following paradox: Euthanasia is legally possible only when the patient suffers unbearably. Only the patient can decide whether she suffers unbearably. But when the patient is no longer competent, suddenly physicians and family members become able to assess the bearableness of patients' suffering. It is completely unclear why the fact that the patient becomes incompetent suddenly makes the physician able to do what he could not do while the patient was still competent. The reverse would seem much more likely. It should be easier for a physician to reliably determine the bearableness of a patient's suffering when the patient can provide the physician with detailed and rational information about her own condition and feelings. Once the patient has become incompetent, this most important source of information becomes either unreliable or falls away completely. The only logical explanation for the paradox is that the paradox is itself flawed. Physicians make judgements about the bearableness of their patients' suffering all the time, not only when the patients have become incompetent. There is actually quite a bit of evidence to support this thesis.

Consider the category of rejected requests for euthanasia. In Chapter 3 (pp. 79–81) we have seen that almost as many requests for euthanasia are refused by physicians as are granted, in spite of the refused requests being quite explicit (75 per cent) and in spite of the patients being fully able to make decisions about euthanasia (62 per cent). In only 6 per cent of refused cases were patients deemed incompetent due to dementia or mental disability. We have furthermore seen that one of the primary reasons to reject a request for euthanasia is the alleged bearableness of patients' suffering. It is only reasonable to assume that the patients themselves did not believe their suffering was still bearable or else they would not have persisted in their requests for euthanasia. If patient self-determination is really the decisive justification to commit euthanasia, these refusals show that medical paternalism is widespread among Dutch physicians.

This assumption is also corroborated by the existence of nonvoluntary termination of life. When the data from the first large-scale empirical study about euthanasia in the Netherlands became available in the 1990s, it was shown that approximately 1000 patients were killed annually *without* having asked for euthanasia. The researchers were quick to point out that although euthanasia requires an explicit and persistent request from the patient, in many of these cases there had been some patient request for euthanasia in the past, or the plan had at least been discussed with the patient. When compiling the data (see Tables 3.1 and 3.2), we gave Dutch physicians the benefit of the doubt and added these cases to the euthanasia tally, leaving only about 400 cases of acknowledged nonvoluntary euthanasia annually. But we also found that the practice of nonvoluntary euthanasia far exceeds that which is acknowledged. For example, in 1995 there were almost 1500 cases in which physicians attempted to shorten their patients' lives by high doses of painkillers without the consent of the patient, and almost 9500 cases in which physicians decided to withhold or withdraw medically indicated treatments without the patient's agreement, again in an attempt to shorten the patient's life. Altogether, Dutch physicians who were caring for dying patients in 1995 decided in almost one out of every eight times to shorten the patient's life without a request from or discussion with the patient.

As pointed out earlier, by definition euthanasia requires an explicit and persistent request from the patient. So even if patients are incompetent and no longer able to ask for euthanasia, this cannot justify euthanasia. Without a request, there is simply no euthanasia. In all of these cases, physicians decided themselves that death was the best way to go, as 15 per cent of them forthrightly admitted. The reasons given by physicians who ended their patients' lives without an explicit request are also noteworthy. Of physicians 30 per cent believed they knew that the patient would have wanted this, even though the patient had not asked for it. One has to wonder how they could pass such a judgement. Four of the other reasons given underscored this kind of paternalistic reasoning about patients' presumed best interests: Prevent further suffering or undignified situation (9 per cent); prevent unnecessary prolonging (33 per cent); no prospect for improvement (44 per cent); further medical intervention was useless (67 per cent).

Not only did the attending physicians make judgements about the quality of life for these patients, but so did the colleagues they consulted, the nursing staff, the patients' family members, and ultimately the prosecutors who decided to dismiss or the judges who imposed a probationary punishment only. As discussed earlier, even the physicians who were prosecuted for murder because they ended their patient's life without a request from the patient herself have never been sent to jail. Several times the courts have imposed imprisonment, but they have always reversed the sentence into probationary imprisonment only. Sometimes the courts acquitted the physician altogether. In doing so, they confirmed that the physicians involved made the right decision.

The Dutch euthanasia debate started in the late 1960s when Van den Berg attacked the power of medicine and the paternalism of Dutch physicians who refused to let go of patients, forcing them to undergo medical treatments they did not want. He ended his pamphlet with the claim that decisions about life-extending medical treatments should always be the patient's. In this light, it is strange that all of the exemplary cases used by Van den Berg to illustrate his defence of euthanasia actually are not euthanasia or even PAS cases. They are all cases of forgoing futile medical treatment or nonvoluntary termination of life. We now know why this is not really strange or inconsistent. His was not a radical defence of respect for patient autonomy, including patient requests for euthanasia or PAS. Rather, Van den Berg was worried about the prevailing medical ethos in which the extension of life was justified at all cost, even if the resulting quality of life was very poor. If medicine creates lives not worth living, it should also be ready to let go of or even end such lives. He simply surmised that patients in these conditions will want their suffering to end. Hence, his proposal affirmed patient autonomy. But even if a patient in such a condition cannot express her will, the physician is still justified in ending her life because her life is not worth living any longer. It does not matter that the patient cannot attest to that fact herself.

The statistics about the present practice of euthanasia suggests that Dutch physicians, or at least the minority of Dutch physicians who are actively involved in MPD, still think along the same lines. Euthanasia and PAS are justified not because these practices realize the patient's request for a medically procured death. Rather, procuring death is justified because these patients' quality of life has become so poor that being alive is worse than being dead. A patient request for euthanasia or PAS only confirms this medical assessment of her quality of life. This explains why a patient request for euthanasia is *not* granted when the physician believes that her life is still worth living, even if the patient is competent and persists in her request. It also explains why the practice of voluntary MPD is only slightly more common than nonvoluntary MPD (15.2 per cent and 11.3 per cent respectively of all physician decisions regarding end-of-life care in 2001; see

Table 3.3). In technical terms, patient autonomy is neither a sufficient nor necessary condition for MPD; but a poor quality of life is both a necessary and sufficient condition.

Shifts in argumentation

We have seen that euthanasia and PAS are generally justified in terms of the patient's freedom of choice. Patient choice has even been made part of the definition of euthanasia such that nonvoluntary euthanasia does not exist in the Netherlands. This liberalist defence of euthanasia fits the broader social context. The Netherlands prides itself on its liberal society and its political culture of tolerance. No single political party ever gains an absolute majority in parliamentary elections and hence government is always a matter of coalitions, negotiations and pragmatism. The state must respect the value pluralism that characterizes the country and hence accommodate as much diverse behaviour as possible. The country was one of the first in western Europe to legalize abortion. It is widely known for its liberal stance on drugs and prostitution, gay marriage and a free market. The recent legalization of euthanasia and PAS is but one more example of state-sanctioned tolerance of the freedom of patients and their physicians to determine their own course of life and moment of death.

The same kind of tolerance is expected of the other major societal force, that is the churches. In fact, there is no fundamental separation of state and church. For example, schools and health-care institutions can be both religiously affiliated and state supported. But these institutions are there-fore also expected to accommodate the religious pluralism and agnosticism so widespread in Dutch society. Only a minority of the Dutch population still practises their religion. Thus, when a hospital or nursing clinic tries to enforce an institutional prohibition of euthanasia, this is quickly seen as intolerance of diversity. Physicians who disregard such an institutional policy are frequently lauded instead of scorned, at least in the popular media. But on closer inspection, the patient's freedom of choice turns out not to be a decisive factor in the practice of euthanasia; rather, patients' quality of life is. The argument for patient autonomy is but a handmaiden in the debate. Or at a very minimum, one must conclude that the defence of euthanasia continues to shift back and forth from an appeal to respect for patient autonomy to the poor quality of patients' remaining time of life.

If it was all about respect for the freedom of choice of the individual who wishes to die, there would be no lead role for the physician. Anybody who is chosen by the person seeking death, and who himself chooses to partake, should be able to engage in euthanasia. The fact that physicians have been given the lead role underscores that euthanasia is not foremost a matter of patient's freedom of choice, but of her quality of life. As guardians of our health and well-being, trained to diagnose and prognosticate our illnesses, handicaps, and other affronts against our quality of life, physicians have assumed the task of determining whether the patient's quality of life still suffices to continue living. Many Dutch physicians who engage in euthanasia claim that it is actually their obligation to perform euthanasia when the patient requests it. This obligation on the part of the physician is not grounded in a positive claim right or entitlement on the part of the patient to have euthanasia. The patient cannot demand euthanasia. Rather, the physician must provide euthanasia because that is what a 'good' physician would do. Euthanasia is part and parcel of the professional role of the physician. Says one physician: 'There are also groups of physicians and lay persons here in Holland who say that euthanasia is not different from murder, and contradicts the role of the physicians which is to cure and heal. As family physicians we are more patient-centered and less doctor-centered. I believe our most important duty is to provide our patients with the help they want, not just the help we want to give. Granting a patient's wish for euthanasia is the last help we can offer in that person's life and to deny that request diminishes what it means to be a doctor.'[204] Or in the words of the former Dutch Minister of Health: 'The doctor who, in such a situation, grants the patient request acts as the healer "par excellence".'[205]

We have also seen that this lead role in the euthanasia debate and practice in reality is only assumed by a minority of Dutch physicians. The majority never practises euthanasia or PAS, or does so very rarely. But this minority, supported by the Royal Dutch Medical Association, nevertheless has been able to change the socio-political climate such that principled opposition to euthanasia and PAS has become politically incorrect.

The resulting non-critical stance towards euthanasia and PAS has allowed for the practice of euthanasia to shift and expand far beyond the initial and paradigmatic case of a terminally ill patient with metastatic cancer and severe pain that cannot be relieved, who is competent and consistently asks for euthanasia, and finally, days before her natural death would have occurred anyway, is euthanized. The first condition to go (in the early 1980s) was the requirement that patients be terminally ill. The Royal Dutch Medical Association argued against it[206] and the courts disregarded it (see Table 3.4). The requirement of a somatic illness was discarded in the 1990s. When psychiatrist Dr Chabot had assisted in the suicide of one of his patients, the Assen District Court on 21 April 1993 stated: 'At issue is whether the suffering of Mrs B was *unbearable and prospectless* irrespective (mental) illness. ... The *cause* of that suffering – whether illness or otherwise – is irrelevant here' (italics in the original verdict). The Supreme Court later confirmed this view.

Although the number of cases in which a physician grants the wish for euthanasia/PAS from a psychiatric patient remains very small, the medical, legal and social acceptance of this expansion is significant. Indeed, it paved the way for yet another shift. Growing old has itself become a justification for euthanasia. When one of the Regional Review Committees found that a physician should not have given in to the request for euthanasia because there were still reasonable alternatives, the prosecutors nevertheless decided to dismiss the case because of the advanced age of the patient. The recent case of Mr Brongersma is also indicative of this trend. He was 86 years old, had no physical or mental ailments, but was tired of living. He experienced his life as unbearable and an unacceptable source of suffering, and hence requested lethal medications from his family practitioner, which he ingested two weeks later. The District Court of Haarlem concluded in October 2000 that the physician's assistance in suicide had been justified (see Chapter 4, p. 118)

However, the prosecutor in the Brongersma case appealed. The High Court (6 December 2001) acknowledged that the Supreme Court in the case of Dr Chabot had stated that the source of suffering was not decisive. But this statement should not be taken out of context, and that context was a medical context. Senator Brongersma's suffering may have been unbearable, but this judgement on the part of the family physician had been a matter of empathic understanding and was not based on a medical-professional assessment. Since the source of his suffering was neither somatic nor mental, the physician could not have concluded that it was beyond prospect because a physician's expertise is limited to medical conditions only. He should have referred the patient to a non-medical professional, or at least urged Senator Brongersma to do so. With its verdict, the High Court appears to have called a halt to the ever-expanding set of justifications for euthanasia. The patient's suffering has to have some medical cause in order to justify euthanasia or PAS. On 24 December 2002, the Supreme Court reinforced this line of reasoning: There should be some kind of medical condition explaining the suffering of the patient in order to justify euthanasia and assisted suicide.

Summarizing, we can conclude that the ethical debate about euthanasia is driven not first and foremost by a deontological concern about the rights of patients and the professional duties that bind physicians. When in 1969 Van den Berg advocated in favour of euthanasia, he was not primarily concerned about the ever-looming conflict between the physician's duty to protect life and the patient's right to consent or refuse life-sustaining medical treatment. Rather, he was concerned about the changing nature and goals of medical practice in the twentieth century. The Dutch courts time and again have allowed the legal and absolute prohibition against homicide, even at the victim's request, to be superseded by the standards of clinical medicine and the prevailing norms of medical ethics. At its core, the euthanasia debate is not about patient autonomy, but about human suffering and quality of life.

These are complex issues. They are also dangerous because there is always the risk that judgements about suffering and quality of life begin to imply judgements about dignity and the value of life. Proponents of euthanasia do not like to admit that quality of life judgements play a major role in the debate because this is exactly what links the present debate to the euthanasia debate from the early twentieth century. It seems safer only to talk about patient autonomy because there is no such linkage to earlier debates. We wish to caution against such burying of one's head in the sand. It allows prevailing opinions and discriminatory biases to direct the practice of euthanasia, defying any and all public debate, evaluation and critique. If the practice of euthanasia and PAS is foremost about medicine's role vis-à-vis patients' quality of life, let us at least be honest and debate this very issue frankly.

6   Lessons to be learned

Introduction

In 1952, the judges of the District Court of Utrecht issued a guilty verdict. It limited the imposed penalty to a probationary sentence of one year's imprisonment, but only because this was the first euthanasia case in the Netherlands. Half a century later, there appears to be a cultural bias in favour of euthanasia. Renowned columnist Karin Spaink has published a paperback about her quest to find drugs to end her life. Her conclusion: death is never sweet but suicide can be courageous.[207] Dr Borst, the Minister of Healthcare under whose tenure euthanasia was legalized, considered it a major victory. Admitting it is not something to be celebrated, she nevertheless concluded: 'It's fabulous that we have achieved this.'[208] Referring to the 20,000 protesters assembled around the parliamentary building at the time of the debate in the Senate, she commented: 'People with such opinions I have unfortunately lost all contact with.'[209]

This bias in favour of euthanasia has frustrated a critical analysis of euthanasia practice. Criticism is rarely taken seriously. Griffiths and colleagues dismiss the studies by Gomez and Hendin as unreliable and give as one of the prime reasons that they were done by non-Dutchmen.[210] Clinical alternatives advocated abroad such as forgoing treatment and providing adequate palliative care are rejected as 'sanctimonious', a form of 'soothing one's conscience'.[211] Jonquière is convinced that knowledge about the Dutch practice of euthanasia is hard to find abroad.[212] Rather than the Dutch, it is the foreigners who are wrong. Former Prime Minister Kok ordered the Dutch embassies to start a PR campaign to rectify the misperceptions abroad.[213] Even the concerns about the Dutch approach to euthanasia expressed by the United Nations Human Rights Committee in

2001 were not taken to heart. The government either politely rejected the concern, accepted the theoretical possibility of the concern but denied the presence of empirical evidence to support the concern, or agreed with the concern but insisted that improvements underway would soon take care of the problem.[214]

Indeed, it has become 'politically incorrect' to criticize the Dutch practice of euthanasia. Conversely, those who have principled objections against it run the risk of being lambasted with fallacious arguments. Former Minister Borst dismisses worries about a slippery slope offhand, as the 'rhetoric' of the Christian Unity Party which drew comparisons with the practices of the Nazis during the parliamentary debates.[215] Professor of criminal law Kelk concludes that any comparison between the Dutch euthanasia practice and the euthanasia practice by German physicians during World War II on demented patients is 'in bad faith' because 'everybody should know better by now', yet he fails to indicate what it is that everybody should know better.[216] Those who compare contemporary Dutch practices with those of Nazi physicians must muster evidence. But those arguing against the validity of such an analogy must likewise show why it is invalid instead of dismissing it offhand or charging those who proposed this analogy with insincerity. Even more aggressive have been the *ad hominem* arguments by some leading proponents of euthanasia. Anaesthetist Admiraal has charged that 'the Christian lobby does not know what they are talking about'. Professor of medical ethics Dupuis (herself a member of the liberal party VVD and former president of the Dutch Society for Voluntary Euthanasia) complained about congresswoman Laning that 'the eternal physician from the Christian Democratic Party in the Lower House ... always speaks up but is not hindered by any knowledge'.[217] Professor of moral theology Kuitert has charged the Catholic Church with slavery only because of its principal opposition to euthanasia.[218]

This defensive attitude on the part of proponents of euthanasia – the 2002 article by Den Hartogh, a member of one of the Regional Review Committees for euthanasia, is a rare exception – has not only precluded a critical analysis of the practice but has also frustrated the development of alternative care structures for terminally ill and dying patients. Both opponents and proponents had always agreed that euthanasia should be the very last option, when all else has failed. Curative and palliative care should always be offered first. We have already seen that the new Dutch euthanasia law likewise requires that these other alternatives must be offered first by the physician for otherwise he may be liable to punishment. In order to advance the level of palliative care, the pro-euthanasia Royal Dutch Medical Association and the opposing Dutch Physicians League already cooperated in the 1980s on the development of a handbook on palliative care. But this is about as far as the agreement and cooperation between proponents and opponents of euthanasia have gone.

During the past three decades, many resources were rerouted to advance euthanasia and PAS. In retrospect, the country could have done a lot more to improve palliative care services. For example, instead of investigating how the insufficiencies in medical treatment and social services that render patients desperate could be ameliorated, the government has focused on researching the incidence and methods of medically procured death (MPD). Instead of developing regional multidisciplinary committees that can assist other physicians to improve end-of-life care even in the most complex cases, a system of regional committees was developed to assess all cases of euthanasia and PAS. Instead of breaking down legal, policy and financial barriers to the development of a comprehensive palliative care system for terminally ill patients, the Dutch parliament developed and debated new legislation to decriminalize and regulate euthanasia. Instead of educating future doctors to provide state-of-the-art palliative care, they were educated about euthanasia. What started as a regional project in the Amsterdam area has quickly been expanded into a national project; so-called SCEN physicians who have been specifically trained to provide consultation in euthanasia cases now operate all over the country.[219] Only recently, a network of consultation teams has been established to provide expertise for palliative end of life. Clearly then, choices were made in favour of euthanasia, choices that could have been made differently.

Jonquière has argued that the Dutch approach is unique to the country because of its legal system and, more importantly, because of its particular history and culture. It cannot be exported.[220] This is too easy a method of insulating oneself to criticism from abroad. We believe the Dutch experience with euthanasia entails many lessons that all people caring for terminally ill patients should take to heart, clinicians as well as politicians, family members as well as judges, foreigners as well as Dutchmen. We suggest the following six lessons.

Medicalization of end-of-life care

The Dutch debate about euthanasia did not emerge in a social vacuum. Thirty years ago, an influential body of social and philosophical literature criticized contemporary developments in health care. The rapid advances in the medical sciences and the introduction of new technologies, particularly in the 1960s, evoked a growing uneasiness with their potentially detrimental effects. These new technologies absorbed too much interest and energy at the expense of attention to the human being as a person. When modern medicine did attend to the human person, it was preoccupied with the somatic aspects, reducing the person to its biomolecular constitution. Commentators began to re-emphasize the patient as a human person and the importance of the doctor–patient relationship. General medical practice flourished by distinguishing itself from the increasing number of techno-logically advanced and hospital-based specialties.

In the 1970s, yet another layer of criticism was added: the charge against the 'medicalization' of society. Inspired by international authors such as Kübler-Ross, Illich and Zola, Dutch scholars criticized the expanding role of medicine in society. Medicine had penetrated and colonized all spheres of daily life. Medical vocabulary was used to explain existential issues, formerly outside the domain of medicine but now recast in medical terms. Medical solutions were offered for non-medical problems. Medical and welfare policies became entangled.

These critical debates quickly focused on the issue of human death and dying, or more specifically the alleged inhumanity of medicalized death and dying,[221] the prevailing attitudes and interventions at the end of life.[222] First, it was argued that modern medicine produces an alienation from our own dying process. Human beings are no longer in control of the final stages of their lives. Hospitals have become impersonal bureaucratic structures where technology is getting more attention than the dying person. As a remedy for this loss of control over the dying process, respect for the patient's personal autonomy was emphasized. Second, modern medicine has a tendency to focus on the patient's somatic condition and physical treatments even if the patient is dying. In response to this reductionism, a holistic, global approach was advocated (e.g. the concept of total pain, and the bio-psycho-social model). Third, modern medicine was charged with abandoning terminally ill patients, who were increasingly isolated and left to their own pain, suffering and dying. Health professionals hence were called in to pay more attention to the social support that patients need in the final stages of life.

The problems that Dutch society began to face in the latter quarter of the twentieth century are not unique to the country. All modern societies have been faced with these issues. Advances in medical science and technology have transformed our ways of dying. The newly gained ability to success-fully treat most medical conditions, thereby extending life, and the advances in intensive end-of-life medical treatment have also dramatically increased the prevalence of chronic and debilitating ailments. A quick and sudden death has given way to protracted suffering and gradual dete-rioration. Many modern patients have lost control over their own death-bed. At the same time, the religious and philosophical frameworks that used to provide some meaning to suffering and dying, or at least make it easier to bear, have lost significance for many people.

Interestingly, in this changing cultural atmosphere three different responses to the same set of problems developed. The first response, typical for the United States, emphasized the need for limiting medical interven-tions. Many hallmark cases, starting with the Quinlan case in 1976, underlined the necessity of as well as criteria for withholding and withdrawing medical treatment. In the same period, a different response developed in the United Kingdom with the emergence of the hospice movement. The early UK literature on hospice care revealed similar commitments to and concerns about a good dying and a dignified death as the US bioethical literature. But the practical solution was quite different.[223] The foundation by Dame Cicely Saunders of the first British hospice turned the dying person into the nucleus of all care activities. A broad concept of health care was developed, aimed at supporting the whole person in all his physical, psychological, social and spiritual needs. The third type of response, the Dutch euthanasia debate, started with the bestseller by Van den Berg in 1969. We have seen that Van den Berg was likewise concerned about the inhumanity of human dying. The Dutch answer to the same problem differed dramatically from both the American and the British.

Why such diversification took place is difficult to explain.[224] But it does yield the first lesson to be learned: The Dutch answer to the problem of medicalization is only one of several possible answers. It is by no means obvious that this answer was the only one feasible for the Netherlands, notwithstanding all legal, historical and cultural differences between the Netherlands and other western countries. Indeed, it can be argued that the Dutch answer is not really an answer to the problem. It rather contributes to the problem. Both the American answer of forgoing life-sustaining treatment and allowing patients to die, and the British answer of developing a support system for dying patients outside the walls of the regular health-care system, break with the interventionist paradigm that characterizes modern medicine. But the Dutch answer is itself a form of medical activism: Death through a physician's injection.

Medical interventions and control over human death

Contemporary proponents of euthanasia commonly invoke respect for patient autonomy as the primary and decisive justification for the decriminalization of euthanasia. Government should not interfere in the private sphere of individual citizens. If patients express a persistent and urgent request for euthanasia, and their physicians are willing to assist, the state has no right to prohibit it because third persons are not harmed by this free agreement between patient and physician.

We have seen that this defence of euthanasia can be traced back to the work of Van den Berg. He championed patients' control over their own lives and existence as an effective antidote against the technology driven power of modern medicine. In this context, euthanasia becomes a matter of empowering patients to regain control and defy the pervasive power of medicine when it renders life meaningless. However, a closer reading of Van den Berg's work reveals that patient autonomy is not the decisive criterion for and justification of euthanasia. It is the overextension of medicine that invokes the need for euthanasia and provides the necessary justification. Van den Berg perceived a necessary connection between medical power and medicine's ethic. As long as modern technological medicine is guided by the traditional ethical prescript to maintain, restore and protect life, the risk of overtreatment and even cruel treatment remains. Hence, medicine's ethic must be transformed. Instead of supporting mere biological existence, medicine must adopt an ethic that supports meaningful personal life. Biological life should only be preserved and prolonged as long as it is worthwhile. If the condition of the patient is such that even the withdrawal of medical treatment does not result in death, active euthanasia is a proper, even obligatory medical intervention, irrespective of whether the patient himself asks for euthanasia. Indeed, Van den Berg alternates examples of forgoing futile treatment with cases in which he advocates MPD. Remarkably, none of his examples of MPD involve PAS or euthanasia; they are all examples of mercy killing, the nonvoluntary termination of the patient's life.

Van den Berg's examples of MPD are all hypothetical, as he underscores himself. In 1969, the 'new ethic' had not yet been accepted. But two decades later, the social context had changed dramatically. A series of liberal court decisions had created a legal system of tolerance. And the large-scale empirical studies between the mid-1980s and early 2000s that euthanasia was widely practised by physicians. But the data also showed that the moral principle of respect for autonomy, hailed in public policy debates as the decisive justification of euthanasia, does not determine the clinical practice of euthanasia. Only a minority of euthanasia requests is carried out in spite of their being urgent and persistent. Conversely, a significant number of patient lives are ended each year by physicians without the explicit request of the patient.

These findings raise serious doubts about the value of the respect for autonomy argument within the practice of medicine.[225] For physicians, the most important consideration and the primary moral justification for euthanasia is not respect for patient autonomy but relief of suffering. If in the eyes of the doctor patients are not in a condition of suffering that is unbearable and prospectless, even urgent and persistent patient requests for euthanasia will simply not be granted. Conversely, if in the eyes of the doctor the patient's condition is worse than being dead, he will consider the option of a medically procured death. If the patient happens to have asked for euthanasia, or agrees when the option is proposed, this obviously makes the decision in favour of MPD easier. But even if the patient is incompetent, mentally ill, demented or a handicapped newborn, or merely hints at the possibility of euthanasia, many Dutch doctors assume that the patient wants euthanasia.

Respect for patient autonomy is claimed to be the decisive criterion, but relief of suffering de facto is. Consistency would yield one of two possible scenarios. In the first scenario, respect for patient autonomy is really taken seriously and becomes the decisive criterion. This would induce a dramatic change in Dutch euthanasia practice. All persistent requests would have to be granted, tripling the incidence of euthanasia. Of course, ending human life without an explicit request from the patient would be ruled out. In this scenario, policymakers will easily agree on very stringent requirements of due care (repeated request, second opinion, documentation, etc.) for euthanasia practice. At the same time, the reasons underlying the patient's request may no longer be evaluated; they are the proper domain of the private valuation by the patient. It is entirely at the discretion of the individual person what constitutes unbearable suffering.

In the second scenario, relief of suffering is the primary justification for euthanasia. Now it is within the discretionary power of the physician to decide whether the suffering is prospectless and unbearable and justifies euthanasia, even if the patient cannot or does not request it. But what exactly counts as unbearable and prospectless suffering? Unlike the former scenario, in this second scenario it will be very difficult to specify the requirements of due care (other than technical and procedural criteria about the drugs to be used and the log to be kept). Yet without hard and fast criteria, policymakers will have to rely on the highly subjective views and values of individual physicians. Arbitrariness in the decision-making procedure looms.[226]

The Dutch euthanasia practice appears increasingly to fit the second scenario. Euthanasia is considered a medical intervention, maybe not a normal medical intervention but a medical intervention nevertheless. The practice of euthanasia, to the extent that it is known, is justified by physicians and in terms of medical criteria. In most cases we do not even know how the physicians involved justified their actions because they refused to report, or failed to label their actions as euthanasia or PAS and consequently did not believe they had to report.

The second lesson is that the Dutch euthanasia movement started as a protest against medical power, emphasizing patient autonomy as a counterbalance. But after 30 years of debate, the power of medicine appears only to have increased because physicians decide whether patients' suffering is so unbearable that euthanasia is indicated, even if the patient does not request euthanasia or, in rare cases, opposes it.

At the same time, it should be emphasized that this growth in the power of physicians is not usurped by all Dutch physicians. We have seen that more than three-quarters of Dutch physicians never practise euthanasia, or only very rarely. A minority of physicians attract more requests for euthanasia; patients in their care more frequently develop urgent requests for PAS and euthanasia; and they are responsible for the bulk of euthanasia and PAS cases. Why Dutch society has allowed this minority of physicians to usurp so much power remains a mystery.

Inevitability of judgements about patients' quality of life

Whenever critics of the Dutch practice of euthanasia dare to draw an analogy with the activities of physicians in Nazi Germany, they are publicly lambasted by a score of proponents, including high-ranking public officials such as the former Minister of Healthcare. The very suggestion that there may be parallels is not tolerated. This attitude precludes a careful comparison between the Dutch approach on the one hand and on the other hand the euthanasia practices in Nazi Germany and, more importantly, the decades preceding World War II. Evidently, there are manifold differences. But there is at least one aspect of Dutch euthanasia practice that harkens back to the pre-war debates in Germany and, for that matter, many other western countries.

We have seen that respect for patient autonomy is widely considered to be a condition for administering euthanasia, but it is neither a necessary nor a sufficient condition. The common denominator in the variety of MPD practices is not the patients' request but the unbearable and prospectless suffering of patients. This presumes that physicians can and may pass judgement about what lives are still worth living when the patients themselves are not or no longer able to make such determinations themselves (because they are newborns, demented or comatose). In addition to the bearableness of suffering, physicians also claim the ability to judge the patients' quality of life and have advanced the alleged lack thereof as a justification for ending patients' lives.

The new Dutch law has in fact granted them the authority to pass such daring judgements. As pointed out earlier, the new law allows for euthanasia on the basis of a euthanasia testament. A patient can write a living will specifying the conditions under which she wants euthanasia. This testament only becomes effective when and as long as the patient is incompetent. The testament substitutes for the patient's express and voluntary request in normal euthanasia cases. But all the other requirements of due care still apply. This includes the unbearableness of the patient's suffering. But who is to determine that her suffering is indeed unbearable? The patient has become incompetent to do so. Therefore, it will be up to the physician to assess whether the suffering of this demented or comatose patient has indeed become unbearable.

But even in regular cases of euthanasia in which a competent patient requests it, physicians cannot evade judgements about the bearableness of a patient's suffering. The patient may claim that her suffering has become unbearable, but the physician must still agree before he assists in her suicide or commits euthanasia. He may not want to pass this kind of judgement explicitly – after all, the government has always insisted that the physician can only assess whether there is still prospect for relief; he cannot assess the bearableness of the suffering. But by granting the patient's request and next committing euthanasia, the physician confirms the unbearableness of the patient's suffering. He cannot convincingly argue that he believed the patient's suffering was not so severe as to be unbearable, yet granted the request for euthanasia simply because the patient claimed it was unbearable. We thus find that judgements by physicians about the bearableness of suffering, patients' quality of life, and the alleged indignity and dehumanization of the patient's condition are inevitable, short of granting every single request for euthanasia.

To make matters worse, these judgements are seldom explicated. After all, official Dutch policy states that such judgements are the prerogative of the patients. Remaining implicit, these judgements may be arbitrary and ever more encompassing. We have seen that the paradigmatic case initially advanced by Dutch proponents of euthanasia concerns an older patient suffering from multiple dreadful conditions who has been kept alive for several years with ever more aggressive medical interventions and now desires urgently to be relieved of his unmitigated pain, nausea and shortness of breath. The empirical data confirm that most patients dying through euthanasia or PAS are indeed suffering from terminal somatic conditions. But the criterion of terminal illness has long been dropped. More recently, the court that judged Dr Chabot affirmed the possibility of euthanasia when the patient suffers from a mental illness only. The Brongersma case could have made euthanasia an option for otherwise healthy people who are tired of life if the Supreme Court on appeal had not decided otherwise. Instead of dying, disease or chronic mental illness, life itself has become a form of unbearable suffering – to be judged by physicians.

Not only did the possible source of the patients' unbearable suffering expand, but so did the degree of suffering. We have seen that 'unbearable suffering', 'pain', 'poor quality of life' and 'no prospect for improvement' were frequently mentioned as grounds for euthanasia or PAS by the physicians surveyed in 1990 and again in 1995 and 2001. All these criteria concern the present condition of the patient. But the responding physicians also listed 'escape from deterioration of suffering', 'prevention of suffocation' and 'prevention of pain'. This proves that euthanasia was not used as a last resort answer to unbearable suffering, but rather as a way to prevent such suffering from even occurring. The prospect of unbearable suffering sufficed to justify pre-emptive euthanasia.

The same issue is at stake in the public debate regarding the 'Drion pill'. The pill is named after a former Supreme Court judge who in 1991 proposed that the government make available suicide pills as a way of assisting in suicide, for example, at the age of retirement. This would grant all citizens an opportunity to end life when they feel it is completed.[227] A complex regimen in which two or three pills must be taken consecutively should prevent people who are temporarily gloomy or demoralized from prematurely ending their lives, or the wrong person from taking the drugs.[228]

The fear of impending dementia is an important motive not only to draft a euthanasia testament, but also to have the comforting guarantee that one has everything at hand to escape from the dreadful existence before it really becomes dreadful. Then Minister of Economic Affairs Andriessen conceded that he would prefer the Drion pill to the prospect of a slow demise through dementia.[229] Former Minister Borst argued in a newspaper interview just a few days after the euthanasia bill was accepted by the Senate, that the Drion pill should be provided to elderly people who had completed their life.[230] The Drion pill constitutes one more expansion of the euthanasia debate in which anybody tired of life or fearful of impending suffering should be able to make an end to his life with medical means. Remarkably, the Drion pill has not received the same kind of public support as MPD in which the physician is in charge. But this may well be precisely because the physician is not in charge. Rather than the patients' own judgement about the unbearableness of being, Dutch society appears to place more faith in the expert judgements of physicians in these matters.

The third lesson to be learned from the Dutch experience with euthanasia is the inevitability of judgements by physicians, in particular about the quality of patients' lives, the bearableness of their suffering, the meaning of living on, the dignity of their being. Except for a very rare exception, there is no evidence that the lives of Dutch patients are no longer deemed worthy of life for economic reasons (although we have seen that the inability of family members to cope is a common ground for MPD). The Dutch health-care system provides financial support and insurance as long as medically necessary. But judgements about the worthiness of people's lives never-theless play an important role in the debate. Health, fitness, youth, inde-pendence and autonomy are hallmarks of a life worth living. Conversely, illness, handicaps, old age, dependence on caregivers and loss of control over one's life are acceptable reasons to end it, preferably at the patient's own request, but if necessary with the permission of family members or without any request – all for the alleged good of the patient. This is the point of analogy between present Dutch MPD practice, and the develop-ments in Germany, the USA, UK and other European countries in the early twentieth century: the danger of making judgements about which lives are worth living. It is a lesson that the Netherlands has resisted learning.

Powerlessness of the law, public debate and policy

But then again, the Dutch euthanasia debate is open and the practice is controlled through a near-perfect system of laws and public policy. It is the one aspect of the Dutch approach that proponents, and even some opponents, are most proud of. Unfortunately, we have seen that this optimistic faith in public debate and legal control is poorly founded. In a pragmatic culture of negotiating solutions for moral problems, it is more important to make euthanasia an issue of conversation than regulation. More energy is invested in deliberation and compromise than in strict auditing of guidelines and enforcing rules.[231]

Physicians are trained to take control and exert a lot of it on a daily basis. They do not easily accept control over their practice by non-physicians. Dr Prins, who was prosecuted for ending the life of a neonate, reminded interviewer Klotzko that he had refused to do his required military service because 'I did not want someone else to tell me what to do'.[232] We have seen that approximately half of the euthanasia and PAS cases are not reported. Indeed, the minority of physicians who practise euthanasia most often are less convinced about the importance of reporting than are their colleagues who rarely have a case of euthanasia or PAS. Many who do report grumble about the need to do so. Those who do not report tend not to consult or keep notes either.

This is the situation after two decades of tolerance on the part of the courts. Only a minuscule minority of reporting physicians has been prosecuted and not a single physician has ever gone to jail for practising PAS, euthanasia, nonvoluntary termination of life, and even involuntary termination of life. Den Hartogh, member of one of the Regional Review Committees that evaluate all reported cases of euthanasia, has speculated that public policy about euthanasia only works if and to the extent that it will *not* impact medical practice.[233]

It appears, then, that the law is faced with a mission impossible when it is expected to regulate medical practice. We have seen that in 1886, when the Penal Code was overhauled and assisting in suicide was entered into the code as a criminal act, no exception was made for physicians. In 1952, when the first Dutch case of euthanasia was brought to court, the court imposed a lenient penalty of one year's probationary imprisonment but only because this was the first case. Four decades later, Dr van Oijen ended his patient's life at the request of her daughters but against the patient's own wishes. He was convicted of murder but judged by the court to be a man of great integrity with honourable motives. To this court verdict, Remmelink added that it must have been difficult for a physician who acted honourably and conscientiously to be found guilty of murder.[234] This commentary by an eminent professor of criminal law, therein later supported by Kelk, another Dutch professor of criminal law, is remarkable since it suggests that Van Oijen should not even have been found guilty of murder because he acted honourably and conscientiously. But as pointed out earlier (see Chapter 4, p. 94), Article 289 in the Dutch Penal Code does not make an exception for people who were honourable and conscientious when they have committed murder.

The fourth important lesson to be learned from the Dutch experiment is the virtual impossibility of regulating the practice of euthanasia and PAS through public debate, laws and policies. Notwithstanding 30 years of public debate involving the medical profession, patient associations, churches, legal authorities, politicians, and the public at large, the Dutch practice of MPD is largely hidden. Many Dutch physicians do not believe they have to abide by the legal regulations that were put in place following these public debates and via a democratic process of legislation. The physicians who practise euthanasia the most are least convinced that they have to abide by the law. The complex procedural system that the Dutch have designed to evaluate the clinical practice of euthanasia may look impressive but does not appear to significantly impact the clinical practice of euthanasia and PAS.

There is little reason to believe that law and public policies on PAS and euthanasia will fare better in other countries. It is unlikely that foreign physicians are more amenable to legal control. In many countries, physicians are probably even more authoritative and exert more control over the organization and provision of health care than in the Netherlands. We conclude that the only option is to change the medical profession itself. Ushering in the Dutch practice of euthanasia, Van den Berg advocated a 'new ethic' in which PAS, euthanasia and even nonvoluntary termination of life would be valued as normal and good medical practice. We likewise advocate a 'new ethic' in which a patient's death is no longer equated with a lost battle; in which the inevitability of death is accepted and, hence, the necessary limitedness of medicine is acknowledged; in which all physicians caring for dying patients must offer state-of-the-art palliative care such that patients are not driven by suffering and fear to seek death. This 'new ethic' requires, first, that physicians are able to distinguish between MPD and palliative end-of-life care and, second, are adequately trained to provide such care – which brings us to our last two lessons.

The importance of distinctions

Ever since the 1969 monograph by Van den Berg, the Dutch debate about end-of-life care has been plagued by confusing terminology and confounding distinctions. Van den Berg himself alternated examples of nonvoluntary termination of life with examples of forgoing futile treatment, as if these practices are analogous. We have seen that the Dutch Health

Council struggled for many years with the terminology, making distinctions in one report only to retract them in the next. Clinicians turn out to have great difficulty in labelling their own practices correctly. Among patients and the lay public at large there is even more confusion. The fear of a protracted and painful death invokes a desire for a 'good death', that is for 'euthanasia', even though that term no longer is used as a label for a good death but only for a death that results when a physician administers a lethal dose of drugs to a patient.

We grant that the ethics of end-of-life care is complex. The distinctions are often subtle and at times difficult to define exactly and explain clearly. But this does not invalidate their importance. It is therefore of vital importance that the following four categories are always carefully distinguished, not only because of their relevance for the euthanasia debate, but also because they have implications for medical practice more generally.

Withholding or withdrawing life-sustaining treatment

In 1969, Van den Berg charged that an overextended medical practice often keeps a patient alive for far too long, even though the medical treatments applied fail to improve the patient's condition and only prolong her suffering. He advocated that in these cases the treatment is ended and the patient is allowed to die. Unfortunately, many physicians still believe that they cause the patient's death whenever they forgo available medical treatments that may extend the patient's life. This is a serious mistake for it is not the doctor who causes death, but the underlying disease or condition of the patient. The doctor merely acknowledges powerlessness in the face of death. It is a sign of humility to forgo futile treatments.

Setting limits to medical interventions will help prevent situations in which patients can only die by asking the doctor to end their lives or to assist in suicide. In many countries, the bioethical debate is now very much focused on non-treatment decisions. For example, many hospitals are developing do-not-resuscitate policies that should prevent cardiopulmonary resuscitation in cases where this intervention is unlikely to be effective or has been refused by the patient. An order not to resuscitate is not an order to end life.

Palliative medical treatment

The foregoing plea for acquiescence in the inevitable mortality of patients, and humility in the face of their impending death, does not imply that physicians always act best when they do not act. There is certainly a place for determinate medical interventionism, even at the end of life. But the primary goal of such care is not the extension of biological life but the relief of patients' suffering such that even the phase of dying remains a phase of living life to the fullest possible. There are limits to what such palliative medical interventions can achieve. As is true of most curative interventions, palliative interventions are seldom perfect. There are almost always detrimental side effects, including the risk of shortening life. Although recent research shows that this risk is probably much smaller than had been feared previously, physicians who administer high doses of drugs in an attempt to relieve pain, nausea, dyspnea and other sources of patients' suffering, in rare cases may thereby hasten patients' death.[235]

This side effect is not to be taken lightly. But there is a crucial ethical difference between such palliative end-of-life care and all forms of MPD (discussed in the following two categories). The physician who liberally but cautiously administers high doses of palliative drugs intends to relieve the patient's suffering. He strives not to shorten life in the process. But since there is no other way to relieve the suffering, he accepts the reduction in the patient's time of life in order to make sure that the quality of the remaining time is optimized. Conversely, the physician who assists in suicide, commits euthanasia, or ends the patient's life without a request, strives to end life. All of his actions are aimed at achieving this goal as soon as possible (and of course in a manner that is least distressing for the patient).

Euthanasia and physician assistance in suicide

The former two approaches to end-of-life care must be distinguished carefully from practices aimed at the patient's death. Unfortunately, the Dutch debates in the latter quarter of the twentieth century focused almost exclusively on euthanasia and PAS; that is, terminating the life of the patient or assisting in the patient's own suicide at the latter's explicit and persistent request. It has generally been assumed that only a physician can do so, although the reasons for this prerogative have never been explicated convincingly. It is also unclear what the implications will be for medical practice in general. If a doctor can end a human life at the patient's request and because the patient requests it, the doctor–patient relationship will change fundamentally. The doctor no longer proposes therapies (to which the patient must first consent before they can be applied). The doctor executes the wishes of autonomous patients. Medical care has become a service on request.

Termination of life without the request of the patient

Van den Berg believed that in certain cases in which patients cannot themselves ask for euthanasia, the physician nevertheless may end their lives. Initially, the existence of such nonvoluntary termination of life in the Netherlands was vehemently denied by proponents of euthanasia and the Dutch government alike. But the earliest empirical study by Van Wijmen suggested that by 1985 roughly 40 per cent of Dutch physicians had already had one or more cases of nonvoluntary termination of life.[236] The 1991 study by Van der Maas, and the follow-up studies by Van der Wal and colleagues undeniably confirmed the existence of the practice.[237] It is justified in terms of relief of unbearable suffering or poor quality of life. But these judgements on the part of physicians in the absence of a request from the patient assume that physicians are actually able to render such judgements. If they can do so for patients who are incompetent, why would they not be able to do so as well for patients who are still competent? And if they are able to do so for patients who are terminally ill, why not in cases where patients are chronically ill or disabled?

The fifth lesson to be learned is that a careful ethical analysis of various medical approaches towards the dying patient and a consistent application of ethical distinctions is important if we wish to develop a care approach that is not directed at the patient's death, but merely accepts the inevitability of death and focuses instead on making that last phase of life worth living.

Towards a broader array of end-of-life care options

It is often said that the legalization of euthanasia and PAS only adds another option to the various end-of-life care treatments already available to patients. In 1992, Dr Admiraal, a well-known advocate and practitioner of euthanasia, claimed that requests for euthanasia were *not* driven by a failure to provide adequate pain treatment – although he admitted that there is always room for improvement.[238]

But the question arises whether the singular focus on euthanasia in the Netherlands has really improved or rather reduced the range of options available to Dutch patients at the end of life. We suggest that paradoxically the commitment to a 'good death' created the euthanasia debate, and the commitment to euthanasia in turn threatened the range of options to bring about 'good death'. And we are not alone in this view. The latest study by Van der Wal and colleagues showed that 41 per cent of Dutch physicians likewise believe that too little attention has been paid to alternative ways of alleviating the suffering of dying patients.[239] The early days of the euthanasia debate were characterized by the image of a 'controlled death'. The significance of autonomy had given rise to a specific approach to death and dying. Death was considered a personal decision, rather than an event that befalls human beings and needs to be accepted as a part of life. The autonomous individual determines when and how death will occur; it is the rational outcome of an assessment of one's own life, the secularized final judgement made by the person himself. According to this image of a 'controlled death', the duty of physicians is to ascertain whether a voluntary and carefully considered decision has been made by the patient.

This image of a 'controlled death' became less influential in the 1990s due to the emerging image of a 'preventive death'. This is the image of a fast and painless departure from life. The Protestant ethicist Kuitert has made a comparison between living and being in a room; one enters through one door and can leave through another. This image of a sudden exit from life coincides with the expectation that suffering will be superfluous and preventable. A good exit occurs while one is still active and feels well, just prior to any deterioration and decline due to disease or ageing.

Euthanasia became the preferred option, not merely when you are suffering but long before you suffer. From this perspective, the option of ameliorating suffering and pain once it strikes appears a second-rate option. Prevention is always better than cure. Why wait until the suffering is becoming unbearable, and then try to ameliorate it, if you have the option of preventing it altogether by means of euthanasia? The emphasis on euthanasia has deflected attention from other approaches to end-of-life care. The first hospice in the Netherlands was started in 1988, more than 20 years after Dame Cicely Saunders established the first hospice in the United Kingdom. Expert centres on pain control and management were established only in the 1990s. The Netherlands only recently developed policies for withholding and withdrawing treatment and identified palliative care as an important health-care activity.[240] The priority that for decades has been given to euthanasia has delayed the development of palliative care and, to make matters worse, isolated Dutch palliative care from developments elsewhere in the world.[241] Whenever Dutch physicians attended palliative care congresses, it was generally to report on Dutch euthanasia practice.

Outside the Netherlands it is often stated that the relative absence of Dutch palliative care can explain the Dutch practice of euthanasia.[242] We agree that it is an important factor but not the only one. As we noticed in Chapter 2, Dutch society is now the most secularized among European countries. In turn, this explains the liberal attitude of Dutch society and its government in moral matters in general, and the pervasive advocacy of euthanasia and PAS among Dutch physicians. Vice versa, the Dutch euthanasia policy is not the only factor that explains the virtual absence of palliative care. Health policy (aimed at the reduction of the number of institutional beds and at curbing rising health-care costs), the organization of the health-care system (with many nursing homes), and the good quality and accessibility of health care in general have probably also contributed to the relative absence of palliative care in the Netherlands.[243]

The good news in all of this is that the Dutch focus on euthanasia has not completely stifled the development of palliative care alternatives. Palliative care can be defined as 'the study and management of patients with active, progressive, far-advanced disease for whom the prognosis is limited and the focus of care is quality of life'.[244] It arose out of the modern hospice movement that originated in 1967 with the foundation of St Christopher's Hospice and adopted the hospice philosophy that care should be aimed at supporting the whole person in all his physical, psychological, social and spiritual needs. Patients must become partners in care. Loved ones, and not merely family members, must be involved. Extension of life is never the primary goal, but death is not intentionally hastened either. Life-prolonging treatment that is potentially harmful for the well-being of terminal patients and that makes the acceptance of their situation more difficult, is deemed futile. But intentionally hastening death is considered dangerous and unnecessary since patients' requests for euthanasia are often ambivalent and preventable in the context of good palliative care.

There are only sparse data available about the effectiveness of preventing euthanasia through palliative care even though one-third of Dutch physicians believe it can.[245] Of the 3200 patients euthanized in 1995, 88 per cent were receiving medical treatment aimed at palliation.[246] Yet in 83 per cent of all cases the euthanizing physician stated that treatment alternatives were no longer available. This would suggest that the palliative interventions had failed for almost all of these patients. The suffering of the patients could no longer be relieved and had become unbearable. But a 1998 study by Zylicz and Janssens has yielded very different findings. Among 450 patients referred to Hospice Rozenheuvel in a period of three-and-a-half years, 28 per cent made an explicit request for euthanasia, usually at the first meeting with the hospice physician. But only two patients persisted in their wish and were eventually transferred to the hospital to undergo euthanasia. The main motive for the majority of patients to request euthanasia appeared to be fear of deterioration, dependency and pain. These patients had often had poor experiences in the past. They had been given the frightening message that nothing more could be done, suggesting there was no hope of relief. But once they were reassured that symptoms could be controlled and had experienced that their suffering could in fact be relieved by expert care, the need for euthanasia subsequently subsided in almost all cases. What can explain this stark contrast other than a difference in palliative care expertise on the part of the physicians involved?

Precisely at this point, there are indications that change is in the air. Palliative expertise is rapidly developing and disseminating among physicians. Expanding networks of regional and local consultation teams have been established. Dutch palliative care journals and textbooks have been launched, professional societies founded, and the number of professional training programmes and educational seminars and courses is multiplying every year. Palliative care has also become the explicit goal of health policy.[247] An explorative study in 1997 identified 6 in-patient hospices and 29 palliative care units in nursing homes and hospitals in the Netherlands.[248] By 2002, a further increase had taken place: 22 low care hospices (mainly run by volunteers), 12 high care hospices (with palliative care specialists), palliative care units in 40 nursing homes (from a total of 330 nursing homes in the country), and 2 more such units in hospitals.[249]

The Dutch palliative care approach differs from the British hospice movement in two regards. First, active hastening of death is not excluded, reflecting the legalization of euthanasia and PAS. Second, independent hospices are not promoted. Instead, they are encouraged to affiliate with hospitals. University medical centres have acquired a leading role in coordinating the provision of palliative care in particular regions and in developing research and teaching programmes. This drive towards integration is due in part to the existence of an extensive system of nursing clinics throughout the country. Nursing clinic physicians have argued that they have been providing palliative care for decades, claiming there is no need for separate hospices. Special units for palliative care have been established in many nursing clinics to underscore the need for new organizational approaches but within existing institutions. In fact, there is growing consensus that the goal of palliative care is foremost about improving the quality of life of terminally ill patients, and that specific organizational forms are necessary to accomplish this goal. Rather than new institutions, consultation services, networks and expert sharing are promoted. Key is a caring attitude on the part of providers in which the authentic needs and wishes of the dying patient are met.[250]

All of these developments have resulted in yet another image, that of a 'palliated death'. Death can be a good death, not because it is fully controlled by the patient, or a timely escape from the growing burden of suffering, but because it is the appropriate last chapter of the personal biography, always difficult and burdensome, but tolerable and worthwhile. Medical professionals must provide the best expertise available to make the quality of this last part of life as comfortable as possible. Even terminal sedation is becoming an acceptable strategy. Not long ago, this palliative approach was virtually unknown. If known, it was rejected because of the implied loss of control and autonomy. It was dismissed as 'hypocritical' because it was alleged to be a form of 'slow euthanasia'. Nowadays, the option of terminal sedation is discussed and explored by many health-care professionals as a viable alternative to euthanasia. The newly emerging image of a 'palliated death' offers hope that new generations of Dutch patients will be able to benefit from the rising expertise in palliative care and the availability of new palliative care services, precluding the need for PAS and euthanasia in many instances.

Appendix I: Digest of Dutch jurisprudence

Krijgsraad North Holland (Military Court) 3 January 1859; WvR 2042
Hoog Militair Gerechtshof (High Military Court) 22 March 1859; WvR 2064,
    2066, 2067
> *Label*: Assistance in suicide; non-medical; death penalty by lower court but
> acquitted on appeal because assisting in suicide was not a crime in 1859.
> *Summary*: A young military cannot marry his girlfriend because the military
> authorities would not allow him to take his wife along to the Indies as the
> father of the bride had demanded he do. The lovers decide to commit suicide.
> He obtains poison from the local pharmacy and they both take it. She dies, but
> he does not (there was some question whether he had actually taken the poison
> himself). The Court finds him guilty of poisoning and imposes the death penalty
> by hanging. On appeal, the High Court concludes that he was not guilty of any
> crime since the Penal Code did not prohibit suicide, nor was there a separate
> article prohibiting assistance in suicide.
> *Alternative source*: L. Enthoven: *Het recht of leven en dood*. Deventer: Kluwer,
> 1988; Chapter 2.

Rechtbank Amsterdam (District Court of Amsterdam) 2 October 1908; Paleis van
    Justitie 1909, 813
> *Label*: Attempt at homicide at the victim's request (Art. 293); non-medical; two
> years' imprisonment.
> *Summary*: Unable to marry his girlfriend, a sailor tries to kill her at her explicit
> request. He uses a revolver to shoot her in the head but, unbeknown to him,
> fails to kill her.

Rechtbank Amsterdam (District Court of Amsterdam) 21 September 1910; Paleis
    van Justitie 1910, 978
> *Label*: Murder (Art. 289) or homicide at the victim's request (Art. 293); non-
> medical; ten years' imprisonment.

Summary: Unable to marry his girlfriend, a young man kills her at her request (or so he alleges). He may have next turned the gun onto himself, but fails to commit suicide and only wounds his leg.

Rechtbank Haarlem (District Court of Haarlem), 24 December 1942
Hof Amsterdam (High Court of Amsterdam), 14 October 1943
Hoge Raad (Supreme Court), 8 February 1944; NJ 1944, 314
High Court of The Hague (dates unknown)

Label: Homicide at the victim's explicit request (Art. 293); non-medical.
Summary: Young couple is not allowed to marry. When she becomes pregnant, she no longer wants to live and asks him to kill her, which he does by strangling her. The District Court finds him guilty of murder (Art. 289) and imposes ten years' imprisonment. On appeal, the High Court increases the punishment to 12 years. However, the Supreme Court annuls the verdict of the High Court because Art. 293 instead of 289 should have been applied in view of the victim's own request. Article 293 in essence describes the same crime as Article 289 except for the request of the victim, which, if present, should lead to a reduction in the punishment. Refers case to High Court of The Hague for final judgment.

Rechtbank Utrecht (District Court of Utrecht), 3 March 1952; NJ 1952, 275
Hof Amsterdam (High Court of Amsterdam), 8 July 1952; Rolnr 524

Label: First Dutch euthanasia case (Art. 293); physician ends the life of his brother; appeal to personal conscience rejected; one year's probationary imprisonment.
Summary: Tuberculosis patient asks his brother, who is also a physician, to end his life. After several more requests, the physician visits his brother in the sanatorium and ends his life with codinovo tablets and morphine. He argues that he could not and should not have rejected the call from his conscience to end his brother's suffering by ending his life. The District Court rejects this appeal to the personal conscience of the physician, arguing that the Legislature did not include a conscience clause in Article 293, as it did for vaccination and military service. In order to send a message to the medical community that this is a serious crime, the Court imposes a penalty of one year's imprisonment, but then turns it into a probationary sentence only because this is the first euthanasia case. The Prosecutor appeals. The High Court of Amsterdam does not believe that it being the first case of its kind justifies a reduced punishment, but accepts the familial relationship between doctor and patient as proof that the doctor was moved strongly by his conscience, and hence reduces the punishment.
Alternative source: L. Enthoven: *Het recht of leven en dood*. Deventer: Kluwer, 1988; Chapter 4.

Medisch Tuchtcollege Zwolle (Medical Disciplinary Court of Zwolle), 1 April 1967
Hof Arnhem (High Court of Arnhem), 25 March 1968
Hoge Raad (Supreme Court), 21 June 1968
Hof Amsterdam (High Court of Amsterdam), 28 January 1969; *Medisch Contact* 21 March 1969, pp. 327–339

Label: 'Versluis' case; forgoing life-sustaining treatment.
Summary: See Chapter 1, pp. 8–9.
Alternative source: WJB Versluis: *Mia Versluis; Dossier van een medisch drama*. Epe: Het Medium, 1970.

Rechtbank Amsterdam (District Court of Amsterdam), 21 October 1969; Rolnr 98–335-I-69-R/6026
Label: Euthanasia (Art. 293) or manslaughter (Art. 287); non-medical; convicted for manslaughter to seven months' imprisonment of which one probationary.
Summary: An alcohol-addicted husband kills his terminally ill wife allegedly at her explicit and repeated request by strangling her. Nevertheless, the Court finds him guilty of manslaughter. The imposed penalty is modest because the Court believes that the man is mentally ill.

Rechtbank Leeuwarden (District Court of Leeuwarden), 21 February 1973; NJ 1973, 183
Label: 'Postma' case; euthanasia (Art. 293); Dr Postma ends her mother's life; Court distinguishes euthanasia from palliative care (resulting in the patient's death) and withdrawal of life-sustaining treatment; blames physician for not first trying palliative treatment and imposes probationary punishment of one week only because of the physician's honourable motives.
Summary: See Chapter 4, p. 99; Chapter 5, p. 134.
Alternative source: L. Enthoven: *Het recht of leven en dood*. Deventer: Kluwer, 1988; Chapter 2.

Medisch Tuchtcollege 's-Gravenhage (Medical Disciplinary Court of The Hague), 8 February 1977; *Tijdschrift voor Gezondheidsrecht* 1978/52 and *Nederlands Tijdschrift voor Geneeskunde* 78/34, p. 1264 and *Medisch Contact* 78/25, p. 769
Centraal Medisch Tuchtcollege (Central Medical Disciplinary Court of Appeal), 30 March 1978
Label: Palliative care does not equal euthanasia even if death follows; physician is acquitted.
Summary: See Chapter 5, p. 142.

Rechtbank Maastricht (District Court of Maastricht), 7 December 1976; *Tijdschrift voor Gezondheidsrecht* 1977/31
Hof 's-Hertogenbosch (High Court of 's-Hertogenbosch), date unknown
Label: Several cases of nonvoluntary termination of life (Art. 298) by a nurse; 18 years' imprisonment.
Summary: 'Frans H' case. A head nurse in a nursing home kills a number of patients with insulin over the course of several years. The District Court of Maastricht finds him guilty of murder and convicts him to 12 years' imprisonment. On appeal, the High Court increases the penalty to 18 years.

Rechtbank Utrecht (District Court of Utrecht), 27 June 1978; Rolnr 882/78
Label: Euthanasia (Art. 293); non-medical; 18 months' imprisonment.

Summary: A 53-year-old woman, who has already attempted suicide twice and believes she is suffering from cancer, attempts suicide for a third time by cutting her wrists. A young man, who had been living with her and considers her his 'stepmother' finds her bleeding. She begs him to provide help with hanging herself. When these attempts fail, he finally strangles her and calls the family physician. The Court finds him guilty of homicide at the victim's request, rejects a plea of psychological *force majeure*, and concludes that this case does not qualify as euthanasia. He is sentenced to 18 months' imprisonment.

Rechtbank Rotterdam (District Court of Rotterdam), 17 April 1980; Parketnr 01805–9 VR

Hof 's-Gravenhage (High Court of The Hague), 16 February 1981; Rolnr 221246–0; Parketnr 018050–9

Label: Assistance in suicide (Art. 294); non-medical; six months' imprisonment.
Summary: After several failed suicide attempts, a woman with several severe mental handicaps and disorders persuades her husband to help. He agrees and builds a suicide machine by hooking up a large hairstyling hood with the gas line. She uses the contraption to end her own life. The District Court imposes a probationary sentence of one month's imprisonment, but on appeal, the High Court changes the sentence into six months, not probationary. It blamed the husband for not involving professional care providers to first examine whether alternative ways of relieving his wife's suffering could be applied.
Alternative source: L. Enthoven: *Het recht of leven en dood*. Deventer: Kluwer, 1988; Chapter 6.

Rechtbank Rotterdam (District Court of Rotterdam), 1 December 1981; NJ 1982, 63

Label: 'Wertheim' case; assistance in suicide (Art. 294); non-medical; probationary sentence of six months' imprisonment.
Summary: Mrs Wertheim, herself 76 years of age, assists in the suicide of her friend by supplying her with Vesparax tablets. By her own account, she had already euthanized her demented aunt some 12 years earlier, shortly after reading Van den Berg's 1969 monograph *Medical Power and Medical Ethics*. The Court acknowledges that public opinion nowadays is more favourable towards suicide than it was in 1886 when the legislature prohibited assistance in suicide. It agrees that in exceptional cases suicide may not be immoral and assisting in such a suicide hence should not be viewed as a crime either. If certain requirements are met (see Table 3.4), the physician may not be liable to punishment. However, in this case those requirements were not met. Moreover, the assisting friend should have known better because she is a member of the Dutch Society for Voluntary Euthanasia (NVVE) which has published extensively about these requirements. Because of the culprit's mental problems, the Court only imposes a probationary sentence.
Alternative source: L. Enthoven: *Het recht of leven en dood*. Deventer: Kluwer, 1988; Chapter 7. Also: Corrie van Eijk-Osterholt: *De dood geholpen. Maandblad voor Geestelijke Volksgezondheid*, January 1982; included in CI Dessauer & CJC Rutenfrans: *Mag de dokter doden?* Amsterdam: Querido, 1986, pp. 55–70.

Rechtbank Utrecht (District Court of Utrecht), 21 December 1982; NJ 1983, 264
   Label: Assistance in suicide (Art. 294); non-medical; court rejects appeal to
   conflict of duties as well as to psychological *force majeure*; probationary sentence of six months' imprisonment.
   Summary: A woman suffers severely from unrelieved pain and wishes to die.
   She asks her husband to assist and he agrees. The attorney argues that he
   showed respect for his wife precisely by ending her life. Since there were no
   other ways to relieve her suffering, he had no choice but to end her life. The
   Court doubts that there was no other way left because the husband (and his
   wife) had failed to get medical and/or other professional help.
   Alternative source: L. Enthoven: *Het recht of leven en dood*. Deventer: Kluwer,
   1988; Chapter 8.

Rechtbank Alkmaar (District Court of Alkmaar), 10 May 1983; NJ 1983, 407
Hof Amsterdam (High Court of Amsterdam), 17 November 1983; NJ 1984, 43
Hoge Raad (Supreme Court), 27 November 1984, NJ 1985, 106; *Tijdschrift voor
   Gezondheidsrecht* 1985/1 *English translation in*: Griffiths, J. et al. (1998):
   Euthanasia and Law in The Netherlands. Amsterdam: Amsterdam University
   Press, Appendix II.
Hof 's-Gravenhage (High Court of The Hague), 10 June 1985 and 11 September
   1986, NJ 1987, 608; *Tijdschrift voor Gezondheidsrecht* 1987/1
   Label: 'Schoonheim' case; euthanasia (Art. 293); District Court finds that
   euthanasia is formally illegal but not unlawful. High Court rejects this parallel
   to Huizer Veearrest (in which a farmer tried to vaccinate his cattle by intentionally infecting them). Supreme Court agrees with High Court but believes
   that there may have been a conflict of duties according to standards of medical
   practice and medical ethics. High Court of The Hague accepts conflict of duties;
   therefore no punishment.
   Summary: See Chapter 4, pp. 100–3.
   Alternative source: L. Enthoven: *Het recht of leven en dood*. Deventer: Kluwer,
   1988; Chapter 9.

Rechtbank Groningen (District Court of Groningen), 1 March 1984; NJ 1984, 450;
   Tijdschrift voor Gezondheidsrecht 1984/26
Hof Leeuwarden (High Court of Leeuwarden), 11 October 1984; NJ 1985, 241;
   Tijdschrift voor Gezondheidsrecht 1985/17
Hoge Raad (Supreme Court), 21 October 1986; NJ 1987, 607; *Tijdschrift voor
   Gezondheidsrecht* 1987/2
Hof Arnhem (High Court of Arnhem), 28 February 1987; *Tijdschrift voor
   Gezondheidsrecht* 1987/35
Hoge Raad (Supreme Court), 3 May 1988; NJ 1989, 391; *Tijdschrift voor
   Gezondheidsrecht* 1989/12
   Label: 'Pols' case; euthanasia (Art. 293); District Court accepts so-called
   'medical exception' and specifies requirements (one of which the physician had
   violated); Supreme Court rejects medical exception for euthanasia; High Court
   of Arnhem rejects appeal to conflict of duties because physician failed to consult; Supreme Court argues that failure to consult does not invalidate appeal to

conflict of duties (but the appeal has to be rejected in this case anyway). Probationary sentence of two months' imprisonment.
Summary: See Chapter 4, pp. 103–5.
Alternative source: L. Enthoven: *Het recht of leven en dood*. Deventer: Kluwer, 1988; Chapter 10.

Rechtbank Breda (District Court of Breda), 8 March 1984; NJ 1984, 504
  Label: Homicide at request of victim (Art. 293); non-medical; one year's imprisonment.
  Summary: After a failed suicide attempt, the patient asks an acquaintance to end her life. The fact that this acquaintance also had other motives to agree to the request is irrelevant. But because of the acquaintance's own mental problems, the Court only imposes a sentence of one year's imprisonment.

Rechtbank Rotterdam (District Court of Rotterdam), 20 March 1985; *Tijdschrift voor Gezondheidsrecht* 1985/44
Hof 's-Gravenhage (High Court of The Hague), 2 April 1987; NJ 1987, 756; *Tijdschrift voor Gezondheidsrecht* 1987/34
Hoge Raad (Supreme Court), 15 December 1987; NJ 1988, 811; *Tijdschrift voor Gezondheidsrecht* 88/13
  Label: Euthanasia (Art. 293); euthanizing physician may not declare that patient died by natural causes.
  Summary: A 72-year-old patient with terminal ovarian cancer refuses high doses of pain medications because she wants to stay fully alert. The physician then ends her life by injecting valium and subsequently pavulon. He next declares that the patient died by natural causes, claiming his duty to confidentiality required doing so. The pharmacist becomes suspicious and informs the authorities. The District Court only fines him for the false declaration, but accepts his appeal to conflict of duties to justify the euthanasia itself. The High Court accepts the verdict but lowers the fine to Dfl. 250 (approx. euro 110). The physician appeals against the fine once more but the Supreme Court once again confirms that euthanasia is not a natural death and this cause of death may not be checked on the death certificate.
  Alternative source: L. Enthoven: *Het recht of leven en dood*. Deventer: Kluwer, 1988; Chapter 11.

Medisch Tuchtcollege Amsterdam (Medical Disciplinary Court of Amsterdam), 25 June 1985; *Tijdschrift voor Gezondheidsrecht* 1985/54; *Medisch Contact* 1986, 951–952
Centraal Medisch Tuchtcollege (Central Medical Disciplinary Court of Appeals), 12 June 1986; *Tijdschrift voor Gezondheidsrecht* 1987/3
Rechtbank Haarlem (District Court of Haarlem), 4 April 1986; NJ 1987, 287
  Label: Involuntary termination of life (Art. 298); disciplinary reprimand; probationary sentence of one week's imprisonment.
  Summary: The 93-year-old lady had been a patient of the family physician for some 15 years. She had multiple diseases, mostly due to her old age, but was mentally still very clear. She had indicated that she did not see any purpose in continuing living, did not fear death, and rejected life-extending medical

treatments. She also rejected euthanasia, believing she had to bear her complaints. The physician believed otherwise. After hip fracture, she refused hospitalization. The physician administered morphine to relieve her pain and she slipped into a coma. The next day, after consultation with the nursing staff and family, the physician ended her life by injecting morphine, atropine and alloferine. The Disciplinary Court imposes a reprimand; the District Court concludes that the wish that life will end does not equate a request for euthanasia and rejects an appeal to Art. 40. Although guilty of murder and liable to punishment, the Court imposes a probationary sentence of one week.
Alternative source: L. Enthoven: *Het recht of leven en dood*. Deventer: Kluwer, 1988; Chapter 13.

Rechtbank 's-Gravenhage (District Court of The Hague), 21 June 1985; NJ 1985, 709
Label: 'Admiraal' case; euthanasia (Art. 293); acceptance of conflict of duties.
Summary: Anaesthetist Dr Admiraal, a nationally and internationally renowned proponent of euthanasia and author of a clinical guide about euthanasia, ends the life of a patient with multiple sclerosis and, contrary to several earlier cases, now decides not to hide his deed but notifies the authorities in an attempt to elicit a juridical process. The Court accepts the physician's appeal to conflict of duties because she was fully dependent on the assistance of the physician, experienced her suffering as unbearable, and dreaded a death by suffocation or pneumonia.
Alternative source: L. Enthoven: *Het recht of leven en dood*. Deventer: Kluwer, 1988; Chapter 12.

Rechtbank Utrecht (District Court of Utrecht), 5 July 1985; *Tijdschrift voor Gezondheidsrecht* 1986/22
Label: Euthanasia (Art. 293) by means of strangulation; non-medical; 12 months' imprisonment (4 of which probationary).
Summary: An institutionalized patient who suffers from undiagnosed pains and has attempted to commit suicide several times persuades a man who is himself frequently at the clinic to end her life. He injects a poisonous mixture but, when unsuccessful, proceeds to strangle her. The Court rejects conflict of duties because the suspect is not a physician and strangulation is not a 'good death'. Because of the suspect's own mental handicaps and the strong pressure exerted on him by the victim, the Court reduces the punishment.
Alternative source: L. Enthoven: *Het recht of leven en dood*. Deventer: Kluwer, 1988; Chapter 15.

Rechtbank Utrecht (District Court of Utrecht), 23 July 1985
Hof Amsterdam (High Court of Amsterdam), 19 June 1986
Hoge Raad (Supreme Court), 23 June 1987; NJ 1988, 420
Label: Attempted manslaughter (Art. 45 and Art. 287); non-medical; 12 months' of which 8 months probationary:
Summary: A stepson attempts to end his paralysed stepfather's life. The latter suffers from several additional illnesses. He had previously asked his family physician for euthanasia and had signed a euthanasia testament. The stepson

had rarely visited his stepfather and had alcohol problems (like his stepfather). After a visit with his mother to his stepfather's nursing home, he consumes lots of alcohol and hashish, returns to the nursing home, tries to strangle his stepfather, but fails when the nursing staff interrupt him. The Court finds him guilty of attempted manslaughter and imposes 12 months' imprisonment of which 8 are probationary. The High Court in essence reaches the same conclusion and imposes the same punishment. The Supreme Court confirms the verdict of the High Court.

Rechtbank 's-Gravenhage (District Court of The Hague), 6 August 1985; NJ 1985, 708
Hof 's-Gravenhage (High Court of The Hague), 12 November 1986; NJ 1987, 609
Medisch Tuchtcollege 's-Gravenhage (Medical Disciplinary Court of The Hague), 28 October 1987; *Tijdschrift voor Gezondheidsrecht* 1988/15
  Label: 'De Terp' case. Several cases of nonvoluntary termination of life (Art. 289); initial verdict of one year's imprisonment but acquittal on appeal because of a failure in due process.
  Summary: When police officers investigate charges of theft in nursing home 'De Terp' they accidentally encounter some 20 suspect deaths. The physician involved is charged with four counts of murder for ending the lives of patients with a variety of drugs without the patients having requested or consented to these drugs. Three counts of murder are proven but the Court nevertheless imposes a sentence of one year's imprisonment only because of the medical motives of the physician (i.e. to relieve suffering). The Royal Dutch Medical Association responds to the verdict expressing concern that it may actually lead to the practice of euthanasia going underground. On appeal the High Court finds that the evidence on which the case against the physician was based had been acquired illegally (because medical records were accessed by police without proper cause). The physician is acquitted. Finally, the Medical Disciplinary Court blames the physician for undermining the public's trust in the medical profession and imposes a warning for not abiding by the established requirements for euthanasia.
  Alternative source: L. Enthoven: *Het recht of leven en dood*. Deventer: Kluwer, 1988; Chapter 14.

Rechtbank Almelo (District Court of Almelo), 3 January 1986
Hof Arnhem (High Court of Arnhem), 15 November 1986
Hoge Raad (Supreme Court), 23 June 1987; NJ 1988, 157; *Medisch Contact* 432/2, p. 44
Rechtbank Almelo (District Court of Almelo), 24 November 1987
  Label: Euthanasia (Art. 293); unduly prosecuted; failure to consult does not invalidate conflict of duties; Dfl. 1250 fine for falsifying death certificate.
  Summary: A 73-year-old patient with terminal cancer repeatedly requests euthanasia. On 16 August 1984 he ends his patient's life with morphine and a curare-like drug. He falsely marks the death certificate as 'death by natural causes'. When prosecuted, he protests his prosecution arguing that it is already evident and clear that his appeal to 'conflict of duties' will be accepted and he will be found not liable to punishment; hence he should not be prosecuted in the

first place. The District Court rejects that claim but the High Court agrees and so does the Supreme Court, even though the physician had failed to consult a colleague. The District Court of Almelo finally fines him for falsifying the death certificate.

Alternative source: L. Enthoven: *Het recht of leven en dood*. Deventer: Kluwer, 1988; Chapter 19.

Rechtbank Alkmaar (District Court of Alkmaar), 8 July 1986; *Tijdschrift voor Gezondheidsrecht* 1986/61

Label: Involuntary termination of life (Art. 298); non-medical; one year's imprisonment.

Summary: When the parents, both nurses, learn that their one-year-old son has Duchenne (an incurable progressive muscular disorder), the father kills him by first feeding him a sleeping medication (mogadon) and then suffocating him. The Court finds the father guilty of murder and imposes one year's imprisonment.

Alternative source: L. Enthoven: *Het recht of leven en dood*. Deventer: Kluwer, 1988; Chapter 16.

Rechtbank Rotterdam (District Court of Rotterdam), 31 March 1987; *Tijdschrift voor Gezondheidsrecht* 1988/11
Hof 's-Gravenhage (High Court of The Hague), 25 October 1988; *Tijdschrift voor Gezondheidsrecht* 1989/13

Label: Nonvoluntary termination of life (Art. 289) by a nurse; conflict to psychological *force majeure* rejected; ten weeks' imprisonment.

Summary: On the night of 12 February 1986, a nurse ends the life of a 21-year-old mentally handicapped resident by suffocating him. The patient was already severely ill, tube fed, unable to walk and barely able to communicate. Neither patient nor family members had requested that his life be ended. The Court found him guilty of murder, rejected the appeal to psychological *force majeure*, and imposed 12 months' imprisonment of which 7 months' probationary. On appeal, the High Court reduces the imprisonment to ten weeks.

Alternative source: L. Enthoven: *Het recht of leven en dood*. Deventer: Kluwer, 1988; Chapter 17.

Rechtbank Maastricht (District Court of Maastricht), 19 April 1987
Hof 's-Hertogenbosch (High Court of 's-Hertogenbosch), 10 February 1988
Hoge Raad (Supreme Court), 28 April 1989; NJ 1990, 46, 47; *Tijdschrift voor Gezondheidsrecht* 1989/51

Label: 'Baby Ross' case; abandonment (Art. 255) or intentional failure to perform life-saving surgery on newborn (Art. 287); acquitted.

Summary: When a child (Ross M) is born with Down syndrome and a life-threatening duodenal stricture, the parents do not consent to the abdominal surgery needed to save his life. When the Hospital Ethics Committee agrees as well, the surgeon acquiesces in the decision and only sedates the child. The child is then moved into the care of the Child Protection Agency (Raad voor de Kinderbescherming), but its representative likewise withholds consent. The child dies several days later. Although the expert witnesses do not agree as to the probable success of the planned surgery, both the High Court and the Supreme Court agree that there was at least the chance that surgery would only extend serious and unbearable suffering. Hence, the surgeon was not obligated to override the parents, nor was he obligated to make a greater effort towards securing consent from the parents. The same applies to the representative of the Child Protection Agency.

Rechtbank Almelo (District Court of Almelo), 1 July 1987; Rolnr. 1175, 86

Label: 'Stinissen' case; civil case; artificial nutrition can be a medical intervention and can become futile; in such circumstances withdrawal is not a violation of criminal law.

Summary: On 30 March 1974, Mrs Stinissen undergoes a caesarian section. An anaesthetic mistake causes shortage of oxygen supply to the brain, resulting in severe and permanent cerebral damage. From that moment on, Mrs Stinissen is in a coma and tube fed. Twelve years later, her husband asks the Court to qualify the artificial nutrition as medically futile such that it can be stopped (i.e. by him withholding consent for its continuation). The Court concludes that nutrition and hydration qualify as basic human care; however, when the means by which they are administered are predominantly artificial, they may be qualified as medical interventions. The Court concludes that there is no legal or medical consensus as to whether the treatment is also futile. The Court sees no reason to question the judgement of the physician in this particular case as to the futility of artificial nutrition for Mrs Stinnissen.

Alternative source: L. Enthoven: *Het recht of leven en dood*. Deventer: Kluwer, 1988; Chapter 18.

Rechtbank 's-Gravenhage (District Court of The Hague), 12 November 1987

Hof 's-Gravenhage (High Court of The Hague), 23 March 1989; *Tijdschrift voor Gezondheidsrecht* 1990, 42–43

Label: Nonvoluntary termination of life (Art. 289); probationary sentence of one year's imprisonment (but waived on appeal).

Summary: A 16-year-old pregnant girl tries to induce an abortion herself but fails. The gynaecologist agrees to do an abortion at the girl's request, assuming she is about 19 or 20 weeks pregnant. On the day itself, he is ill and asks his assistant to induce the abortion. When a nurse doubts the length of the pregnancy, the assistant re-examines her and concludes 27 weeks. But since the drugs have already been given, which have probably harmed the unborn baby severely, the abortive procedure is continued, but unsuccessfully. When the gynaecologist returns, he orders that delivery be induced and to everyone's surprise a live baby is born. When it tries to cry, its mouth is immediately covered so that the mother will not hear. The chief gynaecologist decides not to provide life-sustaining treatment; instead the child is left in a container on top of a heater. After about 30 minutes, the assistant believes the child to have died, covers it, and places it in a refrigerator to hide it from view. More than an hour later, a passing nurse still hears a sound coming from the refrigerator. Later that evening, the child is proven to have died. The Court finds the first gynaecologist guilty of murder, but only imposes a probationary sentence. The charges against the chief gynaecologist cannot be proven and he is acquitted. On appeal, the High Court reaches the same verdict, but cancels the probationary imprisonment.

Rechtbank Almelo (District Court of Almelo), 1 March 1988; *Tijdschrift voor Gezondheidsrecht* 1988/43
Label: Nonvoluntary termination of life (Art. 289); physician orders nurse to inject lethal drugs; probationary punishment of six months' imprisonment.
Summary: The condition of a hospitalized patient detriorates further after an operation. He is suffering from dyspnea which cannot be relieved according to the physician. Although neither the patient nor the family request euthanasia, the physician decides to end the patient's life and, without consultation with another physician, orders the nurse to inject a lethal dose of 100 mg morphine (the patient was not on morphine at the time). The Court does not question the sincerity of the physician's motives but disapproves of his not consulting and ordering a nurse to inject the drugs. The Court imposes a probationary sentence of six months' imprisonment as well as a fine of Dfl. 1250 for falsification of the death certificate.
Alternative source: L. Enthoven: *Het recht of leven en dood*. Deventer: Kluwer, 1988; Chapter 20.

Rechtbank Amsterdam (District Court of Amsterdam), 30 March 1988; *Tijdschrift voor Gezondheidsrecht* 1988/65
Label: Three cases of nonvoluntary termination of life (Art. 289) by four nurses; appeal of *force majeure* rejected; probationary sentences of two to six months.
Summary: Several nurses at the Hospital of the Free University of Amsterdam over a period of three years end the lives of three comatose patients (through a combination of medications and suffocation). The Court finds the nurses guilty of murder. It rejects their appeal of conflict of duties because euthanasia is not part of the professional role of the nurse. It also rejects an appeal of psychological *force majeure* because nurses ought to be able to bear the psychological pressures of working with severely ill patients. In determining the punishment, the Court considers the lack of expert and psychological support on the intensive care wards as well as the emotional commitment of the nurses to their patients.
Alternative source: L. Enthoven: *Het recht of leven en dood*. Deventer: Kluwer, 1988; Chapter 21.

Rechtbank Dordrecht (District Court of Dordrecht), 22 June 1989; *Tijdschrift voor Gezondheidsrecht* 1989/62
Label: Nonvoluntary termination of life (Art. 289); acquitted because of lack of evidence.
Summary: Without being so requested by the patient, a physician injects potassium chloride into a comatose AIDS patient. Because it cannot be proven that the physician actually caused the patient's death, he is acquitted. Remarkably, the Court at the same time concludes that he falsified the death certificate when he certified that the patient had died from natural causes since by his own admission he could not have been sure the patient had.

Rechtbank Rotterdam (District Court of Rotterdam), 3 July 1989

Hof 's-Gravenhage (High Court of The Hague), 4 May 1990

Hoge Raad (Supreme Court), 28 May 1991; NJ 1991, 789; *Tijdschrift voor Gezondheidsrecht* 1992/11

Rechtbank Rotterdam (District Court of Rotterdam), 23 June 1992; *Tijdschrift voor Gezondheidsrecht* 1993/36

Hof 's-Gravenhage (High Court of The Hague), 25 May 1993; *Tijdschrift voor Gezondheidsrecht* 1993/52; *Medisch Contact* 1994, 48: 1377–1381

Label: Assistance in suicide of a psychiatric patient (Art. 294); protest against prosecution rejected, but appeal of conflict of duties accepted; hence no punishment.

Summary: A 50-year-old patient who is somatically healthy but has a history of depression, suicidal attempts (once by swallowing chlorine, once by jumping out of a window), and at least ten hospitalizations requests assistance in suicide. Her neurologist writes the prescription on 2 October 1985 and mails it to her family practitioner (and professor of medicine), who hands it to the patient on 3 October. She obtains the drugs from the pharmacy the next day and consumes them with a large quantity of alcohol. A criminal investigation is initiated ten days later, which altogether takes three years. The family practitioner protests the prosecution. He argues that it is already evident that he will be found not liable to punishment. But on 3 July 1989, the District Court of Rotterdam rejects the protest. The physician appeals but the High Court and subsequently the Supreme Court affirm the prosecution, arguing that it is not evident that the physician will not be found liable to punishment by a criminal court given that his patient was a psychiatric patient. The District Court of Rotterdam then continues the criminal case and accepts the physician's appeal of conflict of duties. On appeal, the High Court agrees that the physician had acted with due care; however, if such a case would take place at present (seven-and-a-half years later), the failure to consult an independent psychiatrist would not be accepted.

Rechtbank Almelo (District Court of Almelo), 26 September 1989; *Tijdschrift voor Gezondheidsrecht* 1990/5

Label: Assistance in suicide (Art. 294); non-medical; probationary sentence of six months' imprisonment for spouse and assisting friend.

Summary: With the assistance of his wife's girlfriend, a husband ends his wife's life at her explicit request on 1 March 1989. His wife was suffering from muscular dystrophy and had stopped eating a week earlier. This family physician had not been willing to render assistance. However, the Court rejects the husband's defence that this refusal left him no choice but to commit euthanasia without medical involvement. The Court rejects the same defence from the girlfriend, even more so since she was a member of the Dutch Society for Voluntary Euthanasia (NVVE) and hence should have been familiar with the requirement of due care, and as a medical laboratory assistant should have been aware of the dangers of taking drugs without medical supervision.

Medisch Tuchtcollege (Medical Disciplinary Court), city and date unknown
Centraal Medisch Tuchtcollege (Central Medical Disciplinary Court of Appeals), 29
   March 1990; *Tijdschrift voor Gezondheidsrecht* 1990/77
   Label: Assistance in suicide; no disciplinary penalty (because trust in medical
   profession has not been harmed).
   Summary: A patient with emphysema is voluntarily admitted to a psychiatric
   hospital because of depression. When he becomes suicidal, he is committed. But
   the patient persists in his requests for assistance in suicide and the clinic finally
   agrees to grant the request. The psychiatrist requests that the commitment be
   lifted and on 17 July 1984 accompanies the patient to his home where he
   provides him with a lethal potion. When the criminal investigation against the
   psychiatrist is dismissed in November 1984, the Inspector for Health files a
   complaint with the Medical Disciplinary Court. The Court initially finds for the
   psychiatrist, arguing that the patient was competent and his suffering was
   unbearable and prospectless. But the Court of Appeal finds that the psychiatrist
   acted too hastily when he assumed the patient's situation was beyond prospect;
   furthermore, he had failed to indicate why he requested the commitment be
   lifted, had involved members of the nursing staff (who did not belief PAS was
   indicated) too late, and had not consulted an external psychiatrist. However, no
   penalty is imposed because he had consulted other psychiatrists and adequately
   informed the family.

Rechtbank Almelo (District Court of Almelo), 20 December 1991; NJ 1992, 210;
   Tijdschrift voor Gezondheidsrecht 1992/19
   Label: Assistance in suicide (Art. 294); patient with anorexia; appeal of conflict
   of duties accepted.
   Summary: A 25-year-old woman with severe anorexia nervosa (since her eighth
   year) requests assistance in suicide, orally, in writing and on a video taped by
   her father. The paediatrician grants the request. He protests his prosecution
   arguing that he will not be found liable to punishment anyway. The Court
   rejects the protest but does agree that he acted in a conflict of duties because of
   the unbearable and prospectless suffering of the patient (short of forced feeding) and is therefore not liable to punishment.

Medisch Tuchtcollege Den Haag (Medical Disciplinary Court of The Hague), 11
   November 1992
Rechtbank Rotterdam (District Court of Rotterdam), 7 December 1992; *Tijdschrift
   voor Gezondheidsrecht* 1993/24; *Medisch Contact* 48/33–34, p. 1015
Hof 's-Gravenhage (High Court of The Hague), 7 September 1994; *Tijdschrift voor
   Gezondheidsrecht* 1994/65
Centraal Medisch Tuchtcollege (Central Medical Disciplinary Court of Appeals), 16
   June 1994; *Tijdschrift voor Gezondheidsrecht* 1994/49; *Medisch Contact* 1994,
   49: 1507–1510
Hoge Raad (Supreme Court), 5 December 1995; *Tijdschrift voor Gezondheidsrecht*
   1996/14
   Label: 'Mulder-Meiss' case; assistance in suicide (Art. 294) by a physician who
   is not acting as physician; probationary ten-months' imprisonment; disciplinary
   reprimand.

Summary: A 73-year-old patient who seeks medical assistance for his suicide contacts the Dutch Society for Voluntary Euthanasia (NVVE). The Society refers him to a physician who meets with the patient on 29 May 1991. When she cannot find another physician willing to participate in euthanasia, she provides the patient with instructions about suicide and assists when the patient takes the lethal drugs three weeks later on 18 June 1991. The Court rejects an appeal of conflict of duties because the physician was not involved as the patient's attending physician, but solely to assist in suicide. The Court imposes a probationary punishment of ten months' imprisonment. The High Court and subsequently the Supreme Court confirm that the physician's instructions on 19 June (i.e. reminding the patient to put the plastic bag over his head and tie it with a rubberband) constitute assistance in suicide. The threat by the patient to kill himself in some other manner does not constitute psychological *force majeure*.

The Disciplinary Court of Appeals considers this case together with two other cases of assistance in suicide by the same physician, all in 1990. In the case described, the Court blames the NVVE physician for advising the use of a plastic bag (as opposed to state-of-the-art drugs) and blames her for not consulting another physician. The second case concerns a patient who had signed a euthanasia testament in 1974 and renewed it in 1988. In 1990 he suffers a CVA, which necessitated admission to a nursing clinic. The patient insists that she absolutely did not want to live any longer but the attending neurologist refuses to euthanize her. When the family physician after initial hesitance agrees, the NVVE physician ends the patient's life on 17 December 1990. The Court blames the physician for not consulting with the nursing clinic specialists who had been treating the patient. The third case concerns a 71-year-old patient with Alzheimer's dementia who had signed a euthanasia testament in 1980. When he could no longer talk or walk independently and could barely swallow, he was killed at the request of his family members. The Disciplinary Court of Appeal concludes that the NVVE physician had acted with due care when she ended his life on 9 November 1990.

Rechtbank Assen (District Court of Assen), 21 April 1993; *Tijdschrift voor Gezondheidsrecht* 1993/42; *Medisch Contact* 1993, 48: 1018–1020
Hof Leeuwarden (High Court of Leeuwarden), 30 September 1993; *Tijdschrift voor Gezondheidsrecht* 1993/62
Hoge Raad (Supreme Court), 21 June 1994; *Tijdschrift voor Gezondheidsrecht* 1994/47; English translation in: Griffiths, J.: Assisted Suicide in The Netherlands: the Chabot case. *Modern Law Review* 58 (1995) 232–248; Griffiths, J. et al. (1998): *Euthanasia and Law in The Netherlands*. Amsterdam: Amsterdam University Press, Appendix II.
Medisch Tuchtcollege Amsterdam (Medical Disciplinary Court of Amsterdam), 30 March 1995; *Tijdschrift voor Gezondheidsrecht* 1993/35
Label: 'Chabot' case; assistance in suicide (Art. 294) of a psychiatric patient by psychiatrist Dr Chabot; rejection of conflict of duties because of failure to consult; guilty verdict but no punishment. Reprimand by Disciplinary Court.
Summary: See Chapter 4, pp. 116–17.

Note: See also Medisch Tuchtcollege Amsterdam, 30 March 1995 for the family physician who was present during the PAS.

Medisch Tuchtcollege Amsterdam (Medical Disciplinary Court of Amsterdam), 14 January 1994; *ProVitaHumana*, 1995, 1: 25–26
Label: Leaving lethal drugs with patient, resulting in her husband taking them; warning.
Summary: Patient develops lung cancer, resulting in severe pain. About a year after the initial diagnosis, patient requests euthanasia and signs a euthanasia testament. The physician supplies patient with lethal drugs which are to be stored at the house of her ex-husband until she takes them one week later in the presence of the physician. One day before the agreed-upon date, the physician consults a colleague. The day itself, the physician brings the drugs to the patient's house, but the patient feels much better and wants to postpone euthanasia. The physician leaves the drugs at the patient's house on the assumption that they will be returned to the house of her ex-husband; but they are not. Some ten days later, the patient's present husband, who had a history of manic depression, gets drunk and takes the drugs. The Court warns the physician for acting carelessly, thereby undermining trust in the medical profession.

Rechtbank Rotterdam (District Court of Rotterdam), 26 April 1994; *Tijdschrift voor Gezondheidsrecht* 1994/64
Label: Euthanasia (Art. 293); consulted physician takes over case; conflict of duties accepted.
Summary: A 72-year-old patient who suffers from diabetes and severe COPD, resulting in breathing difficulties, repeatedly requests euthanasia and issues a euthanasia testament. The family practitioner contacts another physician who is also a member of the Dutch Society for Voluntary Euthanasia who has several meetings with the patient. In the end, the family physician decides not to engage in euthanasia, but the consulted physician decides otherwise and after eight more meetings with the patient (and family), ends her life on 8 August 1992 with nesdonal and alloferine. The Court finds that the physician, after taking over the case from the family physician, should in turn have consulted an independent physician. Nevertheless, the appeal of conflict of duties is accepted.

Rechtbank Haarlem (District Court of Haarlem), 4 July 1994: *Tijdschrift voor Gezondheidsrecht* 1994/48; *Medisch Contact* 1994, 49: 1575–1577
Label: Assistance in suicide (Art. 294); conflict of duties because of patient's threat to throw himself in front of a train is rejected but no punishment.
Summary: As a result of three consecutive CVAs in 1988, a patient is paralysed in one half of her body. She cannot bear this condition but refuses other therapeutic interventions to relieve her suffering. On 14 August 1991 the physician provides her with lethal drugs which she takes in his presence. The Court argues that the physician should not have agreed so easily to the patient's refusal of therapy. The patient's suffering, even if it was unbearable, was not without prospect. The patient's threat to throw himself in front of a train does not amount to *force majeure* either. Although proven guilty and liable to

punishment, the Court does not impose any punishment because of the patient's pressure and the honourable motives of the physician, as also evidenced by the initial plan of the prosecutor to dismiss.

Rechtbank Alkmaar (District Court of Alkmaar), 23 February 1995; *Tijdschrift voor Gezondheidsrecht* 1995/33

Label: Euthanasia (Art. 294); physician should not be prosecuted even though patient's suffering was mental only.

Summary: The patient in this case was neither terminally nor somatically ill; the source of suffering was mental. Nevertheless, the investigative judge dismisses the case, referring to the decision of the Supreme Court from 1994 that the patient's mental (as opposed to somatic) suffering is a valid ground for conflict of duties. The prosecutor protests this decision, but the Court agrees with the investigative judge.

Medisch Tuchtcollege 's-Gravenhage (Medical Disciplinary Court of The Hague), 22 March 1995; *Tijdschrift voor Gezondheidsrecht* 1996/8

Label: Withdrawal of antibiotics and artificial nutrition/hydration; physician applied due caution.

Summary: A 73-year-old patient with hemiparalysis after a cerebral hemorrhage develops a serious pneumonia. When intravenous antibiotic treatment fails, the treatment is discontinued with the consent of the patient's spouse. At the same time, the artificial nutrition and hydration are discontinued. The patient's daughter argues that the treatments were not futile and she should have been involved in the decision making. The Court reiterates that artificial nutrition and hydration are medical interventions. Although a decision to withdraw life-sustaining medical treatment demands caution, the physician did have extensive discussions with other family members, none of whom suggested the patient would have wanted otherwise.

Rechtbank Groningen (District Court of Groningen), 23 March 1995; *Tijdschrift voor Gezondheidsrecht* 1995/34

Hof Leeuwarden (High Court of Leeuwarden), 21 September 1995; NJ 1996, 61; *Tijdschrift voor Gezondheidsrecht* 1995/57

Label: Euthanasia (Art. 293) by a nurse; conflict of duties rejected but no punishment on appeal.

Summary: On 4 July 1994 a nurse ends the life of an HIV-seropositive patient by administering several lethal drugs at the patient's explicit request. The District Court argues that only physicians are allowed to commit euthanasia. The nurse had not simply executed a physician's order. Although the nurse had discussed this case with the patient's family physician, she had explicitly expressed the wish to end the patient's life herself. The nurse's appeal of conflict of duties is rejected. The Court acknowledges the nurse's sincere motives, but for the purposes of general prevention imposes a probationary sentence of two months' imprisonment. The High Court confirms that only physicians may commit euthanasia; they may not even order a nurse to end a patient's life. The Court likewise finds against the nurse but cancels the punishment altogether.

Medisch Tuchtcollege Amsterdam (Medical Disciplinary Court of Amsterdam), 30
March 1995; *Tijdschrift voor Gezondheidsrecht* 1996/36
Label: Assistance in assisted suicide; charge rejected.
Summary: The case concerns the family physician who was present when
psychiatrist Dr Chabot assisted in his patient's suicide (see Rechtbank Assen, 23
April 1993). The physician argues that he was not a health-care provider for the
patient but acted merely as a friend and counsellor of Chabot. The Court agrees
that the physician was not directly involved in the care of the patient, nor could
he have deduced from Chabot's explanation of the case that the assistance in
the patient's suicide medically was not warranted.

Rechtbank Alkmaar (District Court of Alkmaar), 26 April 1995; *Tijdschrift voor
Gezondheidsrecht* 1995/41; *Nederlands Juristenblad* 12 May 1995, afl. 19, p.
722; *Medisch Contact* 50, 46: 1483
Hof Amsterdam (High Court of Amsterdam), 7 November 1995; *Tijdschrift voor
Gezondheidsrecht* 1996; *Medisch Contact* 51, 6: 196–199
Label: 'Prins' case; nonvoluntary termination of life of a newborn (Art. 289);
appeal to conflict of duties accepted.
Summary: See Chapter 4, pp. 112–13.

Rechtbank Rotterdam (District Court of Rotterdam), 11 May 1995; *Tijdschrift voor
Gezondheidsrecht* 1996/6
Label: Euthanasia; appeal of conflict of duties rejected (for failure to meet
requirements of due care); lack of necessity; no psychological *force majeure*
either.
Summary: A patient in the terminal phase of Kahler's disease explicitly requests
euthanasia, which request her family physician grants. The Court rejects an
appeal of psychological *force majeure* because it is not proven that the physician was pressured extensively by the patient. The Court furthermore blames
the physician for not obtaining a second opinion from an independent physician
and acting solely on his own judgement. Since the physician is liable to punishment for violating Art. 293, as well as for falsifying prescriptions and the
death certificate, a fine of Dfl. 50.000 is imposed as well as a probationary
imprisonment of six months. In determining these punishments, the Court has
considered the opinion of an expert witness in psychology that the physician
may suffer from a developmental disorder resulting in lack of judgement and
self-control.

Rechtbank 's-Gravenhage (District Court of The Hague), 24 October 1995; *Tijdschrift voor Gezondheidsrecht* 1996/13
Label: Nonvoluntary termination of life (Art. 289); conflict of duties rejected;
probationary imprisonment of three months.
Summary: On 18 June 1993, the children of a hospitalized patient request that
their hospitalized father's life is ended. The physician orders the nursing staff to
increase the morphine dramatically in an attempt to end the patient's life. The
patient dies the next day. The physician leaves the hospital and cannot be
reached over the subsequent weekend. The physician argues that the patient
had previously indicated that he did not want to vegetate in a nursing clinic.

According to the Court, this statement is not the same as an explicit request for euthanasia, even more so since the patient's spouse denies that the patient had ever expressed such a wish. The Court rejects the physician's appeal of conflict of duties and imposes a probationary sentence of three months' imprisonment. *Note*: See also next case for assistance by medical resident.

Rechtbank 's-Gravenhage (District Court of The Hague), 24 October 1995; *Tijdschrift voor Gezondheidsrecht* 1996/7
Label: Falsification of death certificate after nonvoluntary termination of life.
Summary: A medical resident is confronted by the patient from the former case the morning after the patient has died. Reading the patient's medical dossier, she realizes that the rapidly increased morphine is suggestive of intentional termination of life. She calls the neurologist in charge, who assures her the morphine was given to relieve pain. She marks the death certificate as 'death by natural causes'. The Court argues that as a physician she should not have relied on the neurologist's assurances when the medical record suggested otherwise. However, because of her vulnerable position vis-à-vis the neurologist, the Court does not impose a penalty.

Rechtbank Groningen (District Court of Groningen), 13 November 1995; *Tijdschrift voor Gezondheidsrecht* 1996/2; *Medisch Contact* 1996, nr. 6: 199–202
Hof Leeuwarden (High Court of Leeuwarden) 4 April 1996; *Tijdschrift voor Gezondheidsrecht* 1996/35; *ProVitaHumana* 1996, nr. 3: 77–85. *English translation in*: Griffiths, J. et al. (1998): *Euthanasia and Law in The Netherlands*. Amsterdam: Amsterdam University Press, Appendix II
Label: 'Kadijk' case; nonvoluntary termination of life of a newborn (Art. 289); appeal to medical exception rejected; conflict of duties accepted.
Summary: See Chapter 4, pp. 112–13.

Rechtbank 's-Gravenhage (District Court of The Hague), 25 October 1996; *Tijdschrift voor Gezondheidsrecht* 1997/32
Label: No entitlement to assistance in suicide.
Summary: A prisoner convicted for murder tries to commit suicide while in prison. He claims being innocent and suffering unbearably. He requests that the state pay for a psychiatric examination, to be followed by physician assisted suicide. The Court rejects the demand, arguing that there is a liberty right to physician assisted suicide, but not an entitlement right.

Rechtbank Groningen (District Court of Groningen), 2 May 1996, Parketnr. 030031–95; online at www.rechtspraak.nl
Label: 'Martha U' case; multiple cases of nonvoluntary termination of life (Art. 289) by a nurse; nine years' imprisonment.
Summary: Nurse is charged with multiple murders of residents at the nursing home in Vliethoven. Only four cases can be proven. The Court rejects argument that the patients were all suffering unbearably and/or requested to be euthanized.

Rechtbank Almelo (District Court of Almelo), 28 January 1997; *Tijdschrift voor Gezondheidsrecht* 1997/44

Hof Arnhem (High Court of Arnhem), 18 September 1997

Hoge Raad (Supreme Court), 30 November 1999; *Tijdschrift voor Gezondheidsrecht* 2000/20

Label: Euthanasia (Art. 293); conflict of duties accepted, but physician may not falsify death certificate (*nemo tenetur* does not apply); fine.

Summary: A terminally ill patient with metastatic prostate cancer suffers severe pain that cannot be relieved easily. On 26 January 1996, the patient is treated with morphine in increasing doses. When this is still not effective, dormicum is administered. The patient stops breathing and seems to die, but unexpectedly after several minutes begins to breathe again. The physician then ends the patient's life (as requested earlier) by injecting potassium chloride. He certifies that the patient has died of natural causes. The court rejects the physician's argument that he does not have to assist in his own conviction (*nemo tenetur*) and hence cannot be required to report euthanasia. The Court therefore imposes a fine of Dfl. 5.000 for falsifying the death certificate. Both the High Court and the Supreme Court confirm that the *nemo tenetur* principle does not justify falsifying documents.

Rechtbank Amsterdam (District Court of Amsterdam), 1 April 1997

Label: 'Makdoembaks' case; euthanasia (Art. 293); conflict of duties rejected; probationary sentence of ten months' imprisonment.

Summary: In 1995, family practitioner Makdoembaks ends the life of a 75-year-old patient with cancer at her explicit request, even though, by his own admission, her suffering was not unbearable and without prospect. Furthermore, the Court blames him for not obtaining a second opinion and not maintaining a detailed dossier. The Court imposes a probationary sentence of ten months' imprisonment.

Rechtbank Leeuwarden (District Court of Leeuwarden), 8 April 1997; *Tijdschrift voor Gezondheidsrecht* 1997/45

Label: 'Schat' case; euthanasia (Art. 293); physician must obtain second opinion and maintain adequate records in order to prove conflict of duties; probationary sentence of six months' imprisonment.

Summary: During the night of 17 to 18 April family practitioner Dr Schat ends the life of a patient in the elderly home Doniahiem at her explicit request by injecting morphine, phenobarbital and insulin. He then certifies her death as being from natural causes. The Court blames Dr Schat for not consulting another physician and only keeping very modest notes (even more so since he is a member of the Royal Dutch Medical Association which has published the requirements of due care many times). Consequently, it now is impossible to verify that the physician indeed acted in a conflict of duties and the Court rejects that appeal. The Court also rejects an appeal of psychological *force majeure*. Finally the Court rejects Dr Schat's argument that he is not required to assist in his own conviction (i.e. *nemo tenetur* does not apply). The Court imposes a six-month probationary imprisonment.

Rechtbank 's-Hertogenbosch (District Court of 's-Hertogenbosch), 31 July 1997;
Tijdschrift voor Gezondheidsrecht 1997/57
Label: Assistance in suicide (Art. 294) of patient with anorexia; conflict of
duties accepted.
Summary: The patient has a 15-year history of anorexia for which she has both
been hospitalized intermittently and received extensive treatment. After both
her husband and mother die in 1993, she requests assistance in suicide. In
March 1994, after one more round of therapy has failed, the treatment team
agrees her case is hopeless indeed, but none of the hospital's psychiatrists is
willing to render assistance in suicide. She is discharged and on 20 September
1994, another psychiatrist assists in her suicide. The Court accepts conflict of
duties because the physician is obligated to do 'all that is possible' to relieve a
patient's suffering.

Regionaal Tuchtcollege Amsterdam (Regional Disciplinary Court of Amsterdam), 8
December 1997; *Medisch Contact* 1988, 53, nr. 43: 1379–1382
Label: An otherwise justified decision to abstain from treatment does not justify
the administration of life-shortening drugs; disciplinary warning.
Summary: On 26 June 1995, a 64-year-old patient undergoes abdominal surgery. Four days later, she develops peritonitis which cannot be effectively
treated. She must be ventilated. Her condition worsens rapidly. A decision is
made to forgo life-sustaining treatment, except for the ventilation (which is
reduced to half). On 29 July the administration of potassium chloride and
dormicum are increased in order to shorten her suffering (and that of the
family). That afternoon, the patient dies from a cardiac arrest. As to the
decision to abstain, the Court finds that the physician acted with due care
except for inadequate notes in the dossier. As to the administration of potassium chloride and dormicum, the Court finds that this does not qualify as
forgoing treatment or even palliative care. Indeed, it made the patient's condition worse. There is no indication that the patient wanted euthanasia. Given
that these drugs were administered to shorten life, the patient did not die from
natural causes as falsely certified. Because of the honourable motives of the
physician, the Court limits its sentence to a warning.

Medisch Tuchtcollege (Medical Disciplinary Court) (place and date of verdict
unknown)
Hof Leeuwarden (High Court of Leeuwarden), 13 January 1998
Label: Assistance in suicide (Art. 294); complete disregard of protocol; licence
to practise medicine suspended for six months.
Summary: A family physician provides the patient's daughter with vesparax for
the purpose of committing suicide, even though he does not know the daughter
herself and is aware that a consulting psychiatrist at the nursing clinic had
rejected euthanasia. He defends himself to the Disciplinary Court by arguing
that the manifold rules for PAS are only a hindrance and he does not intend to
abide by them in the future either. Given that this physician has previously been
convicted for euthanasia, the Disciplinary Court revokes his licence to practise
medicine. On appeal, the High Court reduces this to a six-months' suspension.

Medisch Tuchtcollege Amsterdam (Medical Disciplinary Court of Amsterdam), 4 May 1998.

Rechtbank Amsterdam (District Court of Amsterdam), 24 November 1998

Hof Amsterdam (High Court of Amsterdam), 17 May 1999

Hoge Raad (Supreme Court), 26 September 2000; online at www.rechtspraak.nl

Rechtbank Amsterdam (District Court of Amsterdam), 21 February 2001; *Tijdschrift voor Gezondheidsrecht* 2001/22; online at www.rechtspraak.nl

Hof Amsterdam (High Court of Amsterdam), 3 June 2003; online at www.rechtspraak.nl

Label: 'Van Oijen case'; nonvoluntary termination of life (Art. 289) of a demented patient at the request of family members but against her own previous wishes; conflict of duties rejected because patient unaware of her condition; initially no punishment (other than a fine for falsifying the declaration of death), but on appeal one-week probationary imprisonment.

Summary: See Chapter 4, pp. 113–14.

Medisch Tuchtcollege Groningen (Medical Disciplinary Court of Groningen), 22 May 2000; *Tijdschrift voor Gezondheidsrecht* 2001/7

Label: Complaint against physician for not practising euthanasia with due care is dismissed.

Summary: A physician agrees to commit euthanasia on a patient with ovarian cancer. The patient says the necessary goodbyes to her family on 16 March. But circumstances force postponement of the euthanasia to 18 March, at which date it is not possible again to say goodbyes. A professional aid-in-dying counsellor (who had been counselling the patient for a year) complains to the Court that the family practitioner had not acted with due care. The Disciplinary Court dismisses the case because the counsellor is not an interested party as defined by the Health Care Practice Act.

Rechtbank Haarlem (District Court of Haarlem), 30 October 2000; *Tijdschrift voor Gezondheidsrecht* 2001/21; online at www.rechtspraak.nl

Hof Amsterdam (High Court of Amsterdam), 8 May and 6 December 2001; *Tijdschrift voor Gezondheidsrecht* 2002/17; online at www.rechtspraak.nl

Hoge Raad (Supreme Court), 24 December 2002; *Tijdschrift voor Gezondheidsrecht* 2003/29; online at www.rechtspraak.nl

Label: 'Brongersma' case; assistance in suicide (Art. 294) of a person tired of living; if suffering has no medical cause a physician cannot appeal to conflict of duties; nevertheless no punishment.

Summary: See Chapter 4, pp. 117–19; Chapter 5, p. 167.

Hof 's-Hertogenbosch (High Court of 's-Hertogenbosch), 6 March 2001; online at www.rechtspraak.nl

Hof 's-Hertogenbosch (High Court of 's-Hertogenbosch), 19 April 2002; online at www.rechtspraak.nl

Label: Probable assistance in suicide (Art. 294) by non-medical suicide counsellor; prosecution ordered.

Summary: After the death of her mother, a woman obtains advice from a psychologist/suicide counsellor employed by the Dutch Society for Voluntary

Euthanasia (NVVE) about her plans to commit suicide and the means to be used. This is after physicians have been unwilling to assist because her psychological problems (personality disorder with dependence on others) do not merit euthanasia/PAS according to the established protocol. Several weeks later (1 May 1999), on the first anniversary of her mother's death, she takes the drugs but (possibly due to subsequent emesis) does not die. Instead, her brother finds her on 3 May in a comatose state at her house. She dies two weeks later. The Prosecutor dismisses the case because it is not sufficiently evident that the patient died as a direct result of the recommended drugs. The brother of the patient appeals to the High Court. The Court determines that the patient probably followed the counsellor's advice. It blames the counsellor for not contacting the patient's physicians. The Court orders criminal prosecution of the counsellor.

The counsellor and the NVVE then protest the confiscation of records pertaining to the case. The District Court rejects this claim because the relationship between the counsellor and those who typically seek advice from her (and other NVVE counsellors) does not qualify as a therapeutic relationship proper. Hence the duty to confidentiality (and related privilege of non-disclosure) does not apply.

Rechtbank Assen (District Court of Assen), 24 October 2001; *Tijdschrift voor Gezondheidsrecht* 2002/38

Regionaal Tuchtcollege Groningen (Regional Disciplinary Court Groningen), 19 March 2002; *Tijdschrift voor Gezondheidsrecht* 2002/63
Label: Possible assistance in suicide (Art. 294); lack of evidence leads to acquittal in the criminal court.
Summary: A family physician is charged with providing an 81-year-old patient with 9 grams of pentobarbital. This lethal dose had been requested by the patient for the specific purpose of committing suicide. However, when the deceased was found later and an autopsy performed, too little pentobarbital could be discovered in his blood to prove that the drug had even contributed to the patient's death. The District Court acquits the physician for lack of evidence. However, the Medical Disciplinary Court reprimands the physician for violating several formal requirements of due care.

Rechtbank 's-Hertogenbosch (District Court of 's-Hertogenbosch), 19 April 2002; online at www.rechtspraak.nl
Label: Confidentiality of records.
Summary: The Dutch Society for Voluntary Euthanasia and one of its psychologists fight the collection of records from the Society on a particular instance of rendering assistance in suicide by the psychologist. The Court concludes that assistance in suicide by a member of the Dutch Society for Voluntary Euthanasia does not qualify as health-care treatment. Although psychological treatment in principle qualifies as such, it no longer does when it is aimed at facilitating suicide. Hence, applicable laws that cover confidentiality do not apply.

Rechtbank Groningen (District Court of Groningen), 10 April 2003; online at www.rechtspraak.nl

Gerechtshof Leeuwarden (High Court of Leeuwarden), 14 October 2003; *Tijdschrift voor Gezondheidsrecht* 2004/15

Label: Assistance in suicide (Art. 294); non-medical (suicide counsellor); 12 months' imprisonment (of which 8 probational) on appeal.

Summary: A suicide counsellor provides a suicidal person with a list of drugs and other items to commit suicide, opens and places these goods within the client's reach and helps the client take the drugs. The District Court finds the counsellor guilty and imposes six months' probationary imprisonment. On appeal, the High Court agrees (in reference to previous statements from the Minister of Justice and jurisprudence) that providing generic information and mere presence at a suicide do not constitute assistance. However, the counsellor's actions qualify as 'instructions' and 'preparations for a specific action'. The High Court rejects the counsellor's defence that people's autonomous wishes always trump other values, and expresses a worry that people who are merely tired of living will obtain ready assistance in dying from non-medical counsellors. Since the suicide counsellor appears unlikely to change his radical views, the High Court increases the penalty above that imposed by the District Court.

Rechtbank 's-Hertogenbosch (District Court of 's-Hertogenbosch), 10 June 2003; *Tijdschrift voor Gezondheidsrecht* 2003/61; reprinted in *Tijdschrift voor Gezondheidsrecht* 2004/16; online at www.rechtspraak.nl

Label: Assistance in suicide (Art. 294) and failure to render assistance to a person whose life is in danger (Art. 450); non-medical (psychologist); acquittal.

Summary: A psychologist who works for the Dutch Society for Voluntary Euthanasia counsels a patient with extensive mental problems who wishes to die and has written a living will for euthanasia. The psychologist provides information regarding suicide and drugs that can be used. On the day prior to her suicide, the patient has two telephone conversations with the psychologist to obtain 'moral support'. The District Court finds that neither the provided information nor the moral support qualify as assistance because the patient was fully competent, took all initiatives, retained all control, and was not influenced by the psychologist's input. In other words, the psychologist did not provide any 'instructions'. The psychologist is also acquitted of the charge of failure to render assistance to someone whose life is in danger because the patient evidently did not want to live any longer.

Regionaal Tuchtcollege 's-Gravenhage (Regional Disciplinary Court of The Hague), 4 April 2001

Centraal Medisch Tuchtcollege (Central Medical Disciplinary Court of Appeals), 6 January 2003; *Tijdschrift voor Gezondheidsrecht* 2004/13

Centraal Medisch Tuchtcollege (Central Medical Disciplinary Court of Appeals), 6 January 2003; *Tijdschrift voor Gezondheidsrecht* 2004/14

Label: Refusal of life-saving treatment.

Summary: Following several surgeries in the 1980s, an orthopaedic surgeon becomes a close friend of a wealthy older lady. In 2000, the patient changes her will making the surgeon the sole beneficiary. Later that year, the patient falls, loses interest in life and expresses a desire to die. She decides to starve herself to death. When he inherits Dfl. 6 million (approx. € 2.5 million) the family files a complaint. The Regional Disciplinary Committee concludes that the physician only acted as a friend towards the end of her life and the family therefore are unable to bring their case to a *medical* disciplinary committee. On appeal, the Central Medical Disciplinary Committee disagrees, finding that many of the physician's actions at the time of the patient's death do qualify as medical actions proper. Given the complexities generally involved in such life-threatening refusal of treatment cases, the surgeon should not have allowed himself to become involved in the patient's medical care. The Court issues a reprimand. The Court also concludes that the patient's primary care physician should not have allowed the orthopaedic surgeon to become the attending physician for all practical purposes, directing the patient's care. A warning is issued.

Rechtbank 's-Gravenhage (District Court of The Hague), 30 October 2003
Gerechtshof 's-Gravenhage (High Court of The Hague), 4 March 2004; online at www.rechtspraak.nl
Label: Timely prosecution for euthanasia.
Summary: Two family practitioners end a patient's life (28 April 1999). Upon receiving the report, the Regional Review Committee (30 June 1999) determines that this is not a case of euthanasia because there is no evidence that the patient requested termination of life. A policy investigation ensues, which is completed on 17 October 2001. In its verdict on 30 October 2003, the District Court concludes that the Prosecutor has failed to complete the prosecution in a timely manner and dismisses it. On appeal, the High Court agrees.

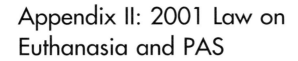

Appendix II: 2001 Law on Euthanasia and PAS

The following text is the English translation as made available by the Dutch government.[1] In such places where we believe the translation is not fully clear, we have placed a note containing our own suggestions.

Termination of Life on Request and Assisted Suicide (Review Procedures) Act

CHAPTER I. DEFINITIONS

Section 1[2]

For the purposes of this Act, the following definitions shall apply:

a. Our[3] Ministers: the Minister of Justice and the Minister of Health, Welfare and Sport;

b. assisted suicide:[4] intentionally helping another person to commit suicide or

---

[1] Available online from the Dutch Ministry of Foreign Affairs (Ministerie van Buitenlandse Zaken) at: http://www.minbuza.nl. Select "England"/Select "Euthanasia Policy".

[2] The Dutch text uses the term 'article' instead of 'section'. This is also the term we have used in this book.

[3] The words 'our' and 'we' refer to Queen Beatrix who, as Head of State, formally proposes and confirms all changes in the Dutch law codes. Hence, in the original Dutch version this bill is preceded by a preamble in which the Queen greets all readers and then introduces the new law text.

[4] The Dutch *hulp bij zelfdoding* literally means 'help with suicide'. The term 'assisted suicide' places the emphasis on the suicide; 'assisted' is only a modifier of the suicide. Hence a more correct English translation of *hulp bij zelfdoding* is 'assistance with suicide'.

providing him with the means to do so as referred to in article 294, paragraph 2, second sentence, of the Criminal Code;[5]

c. the attending physician: the physician who, according to the notification, has terminated life on request or has provided assistance with suicide:

d. the independent physician: the physician who has been consulted about the attending physician's intention to terminate life on request or to provide assistance with suicide;

e. the care providers: the persons referred to in article 446, paragraph 1, of Book 7 of the Civil Code;

f. the committee: a regional review committee as referred to in section 3;

g. regional inspector: a regional inspector employed by the Health Care Inspectorate of the Public Health Supervisory Service.

CHAPTER II. DUE CARE CRITERIA[6]

Section 2

1. In order to comply with the due care criteria referred to in article 293, paragraph 2, of the Criminal Code, the attending physician must:
   a. be satisfied that the patient has made a voluntary and carefully considered request;
   b. be satisfied that the patient's suffering was unbearable, and that there was no prospect of improvement;[7]
   c. have informed the patient about his situation and his prospects;
   d. have come to the conclusion, together with the patient, that there is no reasonable alternative in the light of the patient's situation;
   e. have consulted at least one other, independent physician, who must have seen the patient and given a written opinion on the due care criteria referred to in (a) to (d) above; and
   f. have terminated the patient's life or provided assistance with suicide with due medical care and attention.

2. If a patient aged 16 or over who is no longer capable of expressing his will, but before reaching this state was deemed capable of making a reasonable appraisal of his own interests, has made a written declaration requesting that his life be terminated, the attending physician may comply with this request. The due care criteria referred to in subsection 1 shall apply *mutatis mutandis*.

3. If the patient is a minor aged between 16 and 18 and is deemed to be capable of making a reasonable appraisal of his own interests, the attending physician may comply with a request made by the patient to terminate his life or provide

---

[5] In this book we have used the term 'Penal Code' instead of 'Criminal Code' because the Dutch term *Wetboek van Strafrecht* literally means 'Book of Statutes on Penal Law'.

[6] The Dutch text does not use the word 'criteria of due care' but 'requirements of due care'. The former, much stronger term is the one we have chosen to use in this book.

[7] The Dutch text states that the patient's suffering must be 'prospectless and unbearable'.

assistance with suicide, after the parent or parents who has/have responsibility for him, or else his guardian, has or have been consulted.[8]

4. If the patient is a minor aged between 12 and 16 and is deemed to be capable of making a reasonable appraisal of his own interests, the attending physician may comply with the patient's request if the parent or parents who has/have responsibility for him, or else his guardian, is/are able to agree to the termination of life or to assisted suicide. Subsection 2 shall apply *mutatis mutandis*.

CHAPTER III. REGIONAL REVIEW COMMITTEES FOR THE TERMINATION OF LIFE ON REQUEST AND ASSISTED SUICIDE

Division 1: Establishment, composition and appointment

Section 3

1. There shall be regional committees to review reported cases of the termination of life on request or assisted suicide as referred to in article 293, paragraph 2, and article 294, paragraph 2, second sentence, of the Criminal Code.
2. A committee shall consist of an odd number of members, including in any event one legal expert who shall also chair the committee, one physician and one expert on ethical or moral issues.[9] A committee shall also comprise alternate members from each of the categories mentioned in the first sentence.

Section 4

1. The chair, the members and the alternate members shall be appointed by Our Ministers for a period of six years. They may be reappointed once for a period of six years.
2. A committee shall have a secretary and one or more deputy secretaries, all of whom shall be legal experts appointed by Our Ministers. The secretary shall attend the committee's meetings in an advisory capacity.
3. The secretary shall be accountable to the committee alone in respect of his work for the committee.

Division 2: Resignation and dismissal

Section 5

The chair, the members and the alternate members may tender their resignation to Our Ministers at any time.

---

[8] Instead of 'consulted', the Dutch text demands that the parents are 'involved in the decision-making process'.

[9] The Dutch text requires an expert in either ethics or *zingevingsvraagstukken*. The latter term is not adequately translated by 'morals' or 'morality'. As explained in Chapter 5, p. 140, there is no equivalent term in the English language; the term literally means 'inquiries about the meaning/purpose [of life]'.

Section 6

The chair, the members, and the alternate members may be dismissed by Our Ministers on the grounds of unsuitability or incompetence or other compelling reasons.

Division 3: Remuneration

Section 7

The chair, the members and the alternate members shall be paid an attendance fee and a travel and subsistence allowance in accordance with current government regulations, insofar as these expenses are not covered in any other way from the public purse.

Division 4: Duties and responsibilities

Section 8

1. The committee shall assess, on the basis of the report referred to in section 7, subsection 2 of the Burial and Cremation Act, whether an attending physician, in terminating life on request or in assisting with suicide, acted in accordance with the due care criteria set out in section 2.
2. The committee may request the attending physician to supplement his report either orally or in writing, if this is necessary for a proper assessment of the attending physician's conduct.
3. The committee may obtain information from the municipal pathologist,[10] the independent physician or the relevant care providers, if this is necessary for a proper assessment of the attending physician's conduct.

Section 9

1. The committee shall notify the attending physician within six weeks of receiving the report referred to in section 8, subsection 1, of its findings, giving reasons.
2. The committee shall notify the Board of Procurators General[11] of the Public Prosecution Service and the regional health care inspector of its findings:
    a. if the attending physician, in the committee's opinion, did not act in accordance with the due care criteria set out in section 2; or
    b. if a situation occurs as referred to in section 12, last sentence, of the Burial and Cremation Act. The committee shall notify the attending physician accordingly.[12]

---

[10] The use of the term 'municipal pathologist' suggests that the physician charged with establishing the death of a citizen has to be a pathologist. However, Dutch law only requires that this person be a licensed physician. (S)he does not have to be specialized in pathology. In this book, we have used the term 'coroner' instead.

[11] The Dutch term *procureur* etymologically is best translated as 'procurator'. However, in this book we have chosen the functional translation of 'prosecutor'.

[12] The text of this sentence can be found in CHAPTER IV of this Act, Section 21, under 'D'.

3. The time limit defined in the first subsection may be extended once for a maximum of six weeks. The committee shall notify the attending physician accordingly.
4. The committee is empowered to explain its findings to the attending physician orally. This oral explanation may be provided at the request of the committee or the attending physician.

Section 10

The committee is obliged to provide the public prosecutor with all the information that he may require:

(1) for the purpose of assessing the attending physician's conduct in a case as referred to in section 9, subsection 2; or
(2) for the purposes of a criminal investigation.

The committee shall notify the attending physician that it has supplied information to the public prosecutor.

Division 6: Procedures

Section 11

The committee shall be responsible for making a record of all reported cases of termination of life on request or assisted suicide. Our Ministers may lay down further rules on this point by ministerial order.

Section 12

1. The committee shall adopt its findings by a simple majority of votes.
2. The committee may adopt findings only if all its members have taken part in the vote.

Section 13

The chairs of the regional review committees shall meet at least twice a year in order to discuss the methods and operations of the committees. A representative of the Board of Procurators General and a representative of the Health Care Inspectorate of the Public Health Supervisory Service shall be invited to attend these meetings.

Division 7: Confidentiality and disqualification

Section 14

The members and alternate members of the committee are obliged to maintain confidentiality with regard to all the information that comes to their attention in the course of their duties, unless they are required by a statutory regulation to disclose the information in question or unless the need to disclose the information in question is a logical consequence of their responsibilities.

Section 15

A member of the committee sitting to review a particular case shall disqualify himself and may be challenged if there are any facts or circumstances which could jeopardise the impartiality of his judgment.

Section 16

Any member or alternate member or the secretary of the committee shall refrain from giving any opinion on an intention[13] expressed by an attending physician to terminate life on request or to provide assistance with suicide.

Division 8: Reporting requirements

Section 17

1. By 1 April of each year, the committees shall submit to Our Ministers a joint report on their activities during the preceding calendar year. Our Ministers may lay down the format of such a report by ministerial order.
2. The report referred to in subsection 1 shall state in any event:
   a. the number of cases of termination of life on request and assisted suicide of which the committee has been notified and which the committee has assessed;
   b. the nature of these cases;
   c. the committee's findings and its reasons.

Section 18

Each year, when they present their budgets to the States General, Our Ministers shall report on the operation of the committees on the basis of the report referred to in section 17, subsection 1.

Section 19

1. On the recommendation of Our Ministers, rules shall be laid down by order in council on:
   a. the number of committees and their powers;
   b. their locations.
2. Further rules may be laid down by Our Ministers by or pursuant to order in council with regard to:
   a. the size and composition of the committees;
   b. their working methods and reporting procedures.

---

[13] The term 'intention' in this section does not refer to the intent or purpose with which the physician acts (which is how this term is used in the remainder of this book). Instead it refers to the plan (Dutch: *voornemen*) of the physician to commit euthanasia or PAS sometime in the future. In short, this article prohibits members of the review committees from prospectively advising a physician who is planning to commit euthanasia or PAS.

CHAPTER IV. AMENDMENTS TO OTHER LEGISLATION

Section 20

The Criminal Code shall be amended as follows.

A

Article 293 shall read as follows:

Article 293

1. Any person who terminates another person's life at that person's express and earnest request shall be liable to a term of imprisonment not exceeding 12 years or a fifth-category fine.
2. The act referred to in the first paragraph shall not be an offence if it is committed by a physician who fulfils the due care criteria set out in section 2 of the Termination of Life on Request and Assisted Suicide (Review Procedures) Act, and if the physician notifies the municipal pathologist of this act in accordance with the provisions of section 7, subsection 2 of the Burial and Cremation Act.

B

Article 294 shall read as follows:

Article 294

1. Any person who intentionally incites another to commit suicide shall, if suicide follows, be liable to a term of imprisonment not exceeding three years or to a fourth-category fine.
2. Any person who intentionally assists another to commit suicide or provides him with the means to do so shall, if suicide follows, be liable to a term of imprisonment not exceeding three years or a fourth-category fine. Article 293, paragraph 2 shall apply *mutatis mutandis*.

[*Under C and D two more minor changes in other articles are described to make sure those reflect the changes under A and B.*]

Section 21

The Burial and Cremation Act shall be amended as follows.

A

Section 7 shall read as follows:

Section 7

1. The person who conducted the post-mortem examination shall issue a death certificate if he is satisfied that the death was due to natural causes.

2. If death was the result of the termination of life on request or assisted suicide as referred to in article 293, paragraph 2, or article 294, paragraph 2, second sentence, of the Criminal Code respectively, the attending physician shall not issue a death certificate and shall immediately notify the municipal pathologist or one of the municipal pathologists of the cause of death by completing a report form. The attending physician shall enclose with the form a detailed report on compliance with the due care criteria set out in section 2 of the Termination of Life on Request and Assisted Suicide (Review Procedures) Act.
3. If the attending physician decides, in cases other than those referred to in subsection 2, that he is unable to issue a death certificate, he shall immediately notify the municipal pathologist or one of the municipal pathologists accordingly by completing a report form.

B

Section 9 shall read as follows:

Section 9

1. The form and layout of the models for the death certificates to be issued by the attending physician and the municipal pathologist shall be laid down by order in council.
2. The form and layout of the models for the notification and the detailed report as referred to in section 7, subsection 2, for the notification as referred to in section 7, subsection 3 and for the forms referred to in section 10, subsections 1 and 2, shall be laid down by order in council on the recommendation of Our Minister of Justice and Our Minister of Health, Welfare and Sport.

C

Section 10 shall read as follows:

Section 10

1. If the municipal pathologist decides that he is unable to issue a death certificate, he shall immediately notify the public prosecutor by completing a form and shall immediately notify the Registrar of Births, Deaths and Marriages.
2. Without prejudice to subsection 1, the municipal pathologist shall, if notified as referred to in section 7, subsection 2, report without delay to the regional review committees referred to in section 3 of the Termination of Life on Request and Assisted Suicide (Review Procedures) Act by completing a form. He shall enclose a detailed report as referred to in section 7, subsection 2.[14]

D

The following sentence shall be added to section 12: If the public prosecutor decides, in cases as referred to in section 7, subsection 2, that he is unable to issue a certificate

---

[14] The reference here is to section 7, subsection 2 of the Burial and Cremation Act. For the revised text of this section, see CHAPTER IV, Section 21, under 'A' of the present Act.

of no objection to burial or cremation, he shall immediately notify the municipal pathologist and the regional review committee as referred to in section 3 of the Termination of Life on Request and Assisted Suicide (Review Procedures) Act.

[*Under E one more minor change in another article is described to make sure it reflects the changes described above. Section 22 likewise describes a minor change in the General Administrative Law Act to make it consistent with this new act.*]

CHAPTER V. CONCLUDING PROVISIONS

Section 23

This Act shall enter into force on a date to be determined by Royal Decree.[15]

Section 24

This Act may be cited as the Termination of Life on Request and Assisted Suicide (Review Procedures) Act.

We order and command that this Act shall be published in the Bulletin of Acts and Decrees and that all ministries, authorities, bodies and officials whom it may concern shall diligently implement it.

---

[15] The Act took effect on 1 April 2002

Notes

1. Indewey Gerlings-Huurman 1977.
2. Leenen 1977: 72–146.
3. Muntendam 1977: 5–15.
4. Sporken 1977.
5. Enthoven 1987; Hoogerkamp 1992: 13.
6. Beemer 1977: 30–47.
7. Staatscommissie Euthanasie 1985, p. 26.
8. Van der Wal and Van der Maas 1996.
9. Jochemsen and Keown 1999, 25: 16–21.
10. Meerman 1991.
11. Dowbiggin 2003.
12. Hoogerwerf 1999.
13. Ten Have and Janssens 2001; Janssens, Ten Have and Zylicz 1999, 25: 408–12.
14. Kolfschoten 2003, 361: 1352–3.
15. Available online at http://www.coe.int/euthanasia-report.
16. Van der Wal et al. 2003.
17. Van den Berg 1969, 5, p. 48.
18. Van den Berg 1956.
19. Van den Berg 1959; Van den Berg 1961.
20. Van den Berg 1969, 5, p. 27.
21. Van den Berg 1969, 5, p. 37.
22. Handelingen Tweede Kamer, 1959–1970, 40ste vergadering, p. 1952.
23. Rigter 1992.
24. Ten Have and Clark 2002.
25. Gezondheidsraad 1973, p. 6.
26. KNMG – Koninklijke Nederlandsche Maatschappij tot Bevordering der Geneeskunst 1936, p. 7.
27. Ten Have and Janssens 2001, p. 18.

28. KNMG – Koninklijke Nederlandsche Maatschappij tot Bevordering der Geneeskunst 1959, p. 10.
29. KNMG – Koninklijke Nederlandsche Maatschappij tot Bevordering der Geneeskunst 1959, p. 14.
30. Salomon 1948, p. 30.
31. Proctor 1988, p. 193; italics by Proctor.
32. Menges 1972.
33. Available online at the website of the World Medical Association (www.wma.net).
34. Veatch 1978, 1: 172–80.
35. Mertens 1960, 39: 94–100.
36. Galbraith 1978, 4: 61–3.
37. Orie 1968, 112: 1832–6.
38. Den Otter 1968, 23: 846–50.
39. Ten Have 1995, 16: 3–14.
40. Von Weizsäcker 1950: 136–66.
41. Buytendijk 1947.
42. Buytendijk 1959, 103: 2504–8.
43. Juffermans 1982.
44. Huysmans et al. 1973.
45. McWhinney 1989, p. 56.
46. Huygen 1978.
47. Dunning 1981.
48. Lindeboom 1979, 123: 1610–11.
49. Felling, Peters and Schreuder 1991.
50. Becker and Vink 1994.
51. Dekker, De Hart and Peters 1997.
52. Halman et al. 1987.
53. Dekker, De Hart and Peters 1997.
54. Felling, Peters and Schreuder 1991, p. 14.
55. Becker and De Wit 2000.
56. Becker and Vink 1994.
57. Van den Hoofdakker 1970.
58. Zola 1972, 15: 229–30.
59. Illich 1975.
60. Illich 1975, p. 26.
61. Illich 1975, p. 59.
62. Illich 1975, pp. 149–50.
63. Terborgh-Dupuis 1976.
64. Aghina 1978.
65. Illich 1975, p. 150.
66. Matse 1974: 138–45.
67. Dekkers 2001: 411–31.
68. See for example Ariès 1974, 1981, 1985.
69. Van Es 1974: 59–72.
70. Bruntink 2002.
71. Elias 1985.
72. Kuitert 1993.

73. Chabot 2001.
74. Hilhorst 1983.
75. Kenter 1983, 38: 1179–82; Ponsioen 1983, 127: 961–4.
76. Klijn and Nieboer 1984.
77. Dierick 1983, 1: 1–239; Sporken 1981.
78. Kuitert 1981; Leenen 1978: 1–8.
79. Klijn and Nieboer 1984.
80. Sporken 1981.
81. Klijn and Nieboer 1984.
82. CAL – Commissie Aanvaardbaarheid Levensbeëindigend Handelen 1997;
    NVK – Nederlandse Vereniging voor Kindergeneeskunde 1992; NVP –
    Nederlandse Vereniging voor Psychiatrie 1992, 86: 2–3.
83. Klotzko 1997, 93: 38–9.
84. SCP – Sociaal en Cultureel Planbureau 2002, pp. 162–3.
85. Beemer 1986: 33–47, p. 38.
86. Van der Wal and Van der Maas 1996; Van der Wal, Van der Maas and Bosma
    1996, 335: 1706–11.
87. Ten Have and Janssens 1997, 94: 393–9.
88. De Wachter 1992, 326(2): 128–33.
89. Meyler 1973, 117: 553–5.
90. CAL – Commissie Aanvaardbaarheid Levensbeëindigend Handelen 1997.
91. Hoogerkamp 1992, 13.
92. Legemate 1998, 8: 14–20.
93. KNMG – Koninklijke Nederlandse Maatschappij tot Bevordering der Ge-
    neeskunst 1997, 53: 420–25.
94. Veldhuis 1988, 11: 63–7, p. 71.
95. Gordijn 1998, 10: 12–25.
96. Welie 1992, 17(4): 419–37.
97. Van den Berg 1969, 5, p. 48.
98. See, for example, Gomez 1991, 118(14, suppl.) 469–72; Van der Maas, Van
    Delden and Pijnenborg 1991; Pool 2000; The 1997; Thomasma et al. 1998;
    Van der Wal et al. 2003; Van der Wal and Van der Maas et al. 1996.
99. Van der Wal et al. 2003, p. 49.
100. Thomasma et al. 1998, pp. 411, 422.
101. Regionale Toetsingscommissies Euthanasie 2002, p. 12.
102. Regionale Toetsingscommissies Euthanasie 2001, 2002, 2003.
103. Van der Wal et al. 2003, p. 49.
104. Van der Wal et al. 2003, p. 51.
105. Onwuteaka-Philipsen 1999, p. 45.
106. Van der Wal et al. 1991c, 46: 174–6, p. 174.
107. Van der Maas, Van Delden and Pijnenborg 1991, p. 58.
108. Van Delden, Pijnenborg and Van der Maas 1993, 7: 323–9.
109. Van der Wal et al. 1991a, 46: 171–3; Van der Wal et al. 1991b, 46: 211–15;
     Van der Wal et al. 1991c, 46: 174–6; Van der Wal et al. 1991d, 46: 237–45;
     Van der Wal 1992.
110. Den Hartogh 2002, 26: 232–50, p. 234.
111. Van der Maas, Van Delden and Pijnenborg 1991, p. 60.
112. Keown 1995: 261–96.

113. Thomasma et al. 1998.
114. Interview with Coen Verbaak in *Vrij Nederland*, 10 August 1994.
115. Medical Disciplinary Court of The Hague, 11 November 1992.
116. *Radbode – University Medical Center Nijmegen Newsletter*, 22 April 2001.
117. Thomasma et al. 1998, p. 340.
118. Van der Wal et al. 2003.
119. Van der Wal 1992, pp. 24–5.
120. Van der Wal 1992, p. 23.
121. Thomasma et al. 1998, p. 303.
122. Van der Wal et al. 2003, p. 46.
123. Thomasma et al. 1998, p. 351.
124. Thomasma et al. 1998, p. 287.
125. Thomasma et al. 1998, p. 274.
126. Thomasma et al. 1998, p. 289.
127. Thomasma et al. 1998, p. 276.
128. Thomasma et al. 1998, p. 291.
129. Thomasma et al. 1998, p. 295.
130. Thomasma et al. 1998, p. 287.
131. Thomasma et al. 1998, p. 282.
132. Thomasma et al. 1998, p. 297.
133. Thomasma et al. 1998, p. 381.
134. Klijn, Otlowski and Trappenburg 2001.
135. Van der Wal and Van der Maas 1996, p. 60.
136. Van der Wal and Van der Maas 1996, p. 174.
137. Van der Wal and Van der Maas 1996, p. 61.
138. Handelingen Tweede Kamer, 1998–1999, 26691 (3), pp. 8–9.
139. Haverkate et al. 2001, 145: 80–4.
140. Van Wijmen 1989, p. 30.
141. Arentz 2001, 56: 217–18.
142. Van Wijmen 1989, p. 21.
143. Van der Wal 1992, p. 22.
144. Arentz 2001, 56: 217–18.
145. Van Wijmen 1989, p. 25.
146. Van der Wal and Van der Maas 1996, p. 119.
147. Van der Wal et al. 2003, p. 165.
148. Van der Wal and Van der Maas 1996, p. 117.
149. Van der Wal et al. 2003, p. 168.
150. Den Hartogh 2002, 26: 232–50, p. 238.
151. Concluding Observations of the Human Rights Committee: Netherlands; 20/07/2001. CCPR/CO/72/NET, §5b.
152. Den Hartogh 2002, 26: 232–50.
153. Van der Wal and Van der Maas 1996, p. 115.
154. Regionale Toetsingscommissies Euthanasie 2000, 2001, 2002.
155. Regionale Toetsingscommissies Euthanasie 2000, p. 14.
156. Wibaut 2001, 56: 657–9.
157. Groenewoud et al. 2000, 342: 551–6.
158. Thomasma et al. 1998, p. 297.
159. Van Wijmen 1989, p. 29.

160. Van der Wal and Van der Maas 1996, p. 172.
161. See, for example, Handelingen Tweede Kamer, 1999–2000, 26991, 6, pp. 2, 17.
162. Handelingen Tweede Kamer, 1999–2000, 26991, (5), p. 6; (6), p. 5.
163. See, for example, District Court of Rotterdam on 17 April 1980; District Court of Rotterdam on 1 December 1981; District Court of Utrecht on 21 December 1982; District Court of Rotterdam on 7 December 1992.
164. See also Ten Have and Welie 1992, 22: 34–8; Welie 2002, 32: 42–44.
165. Jonquière 2002, 57: 505–7.
166. Enthoven 1998, Chapter 3.
167. Remmelink 2001, 19: 896.
168. Remmelink 1996, 15, § 2.4.3.
169. Welie 1992, 17(4): 419–37.
170. See also the second verdict of the Dutch Supreme Court in the Groningen case of Dr Pols from 1984 cited on page 103.
171. For a comprehensive list of published Dutch Jurisprudence on euthanasia and PAS, see Appendix I.
172. Klotzko and Chabot 1998: 373–87, pp. 380–1.
173. Van der Ree 2001, 56: 426–8.
174. Van der Ree 2001, 56: 426–8.
175. Klotzko and Chabot 1998: 373–87, p. 383.
176. Weyers 2002.
177. Handelingen Tweede Kamer, 1998–1999, 26691, (3), pp. 8–9.
178. Disciplinary Court of The Hague from 4 April 2001; and the subsequent verdict on appeal by the Central Medical Disciplinary Court from 6 January 2003.
179. Jacobs 1990, 45: 541–3.
180. Van Delden 1993.
181. Thomasma et al. 1998, p. 286.
182. See e.g. Van Delden, Pijnenborg, and Van der Maas 1993, 7: 323–9; Griffiths, Bood and Weyers 1998.
183. Van Wijmen 1989.
184. KNMG – Koninklijke Nederlandse Maatschappij tot Bevordering der Geneeskunst 1984, 31: 990–1002, p. 992.
185. NVVE – Nederlandse Vereniging voor Vrijwillige Euthanasie 1991, p. 5.
186. Handelingen Tweede Kamer, 26691, (6), pp. 37, 80.
187. Gezondheidsraad 1973, 1982c.
188. KNMG – Koninklijke Nederlandse Maatschappij tot Bevordering der Geneeskunst 1984, 31: 990–1002.
189. Gezondheidsraad 1982b.
190. Gezondheidsraad 1982a.
191. See also Supreme Court, 8 February 1944.
192. Press release from 17 February 1995, in: Dutch Catholic Bishops' Conference 2002.
193. Klotzko and Chabot 1998: 373–87, p. 376.
194. Van Wijmen 1989, p. 14.
195. Meulenbelt 1986, 13: 7–14.
196. Handelingen Tweede Kamer, 1998–1999, 26691, 3, Artikel 2.

197. Van Wijmen 1989, pp. 13–14.
198. Regionale Toetsingscommissies Euthanasie 2001, p. 17.
199. Van der Wal and Van der Maas 1996, p. 62.
200. Van der Wal and Van der Maas 1996.
201. Jannink-Kappelle 1992, 47: 845–7; NVVE – Nederlandse Vereniging voor Vrijwillige Euthanasie 1992, 47: 846–7.
202. Welie 2001, 4: 169–83; Welie 2004: 163–80.
203. Interview with Margriet Oostveen: 'Mijn familie heeft een traditie in zelfdo- dingen,' *NRC Handelsblad* from 28 April 2001.
204. Thomasma et al. 1998, p. 372.
205. Borst-Eilers 1992: 55–68.
206. KNMG – Koninklijke Nederlandse Maatschappij tot Bevordering der Ge- neeskunst 1984, 31: 990–1002.
207. Spaink 2001.
208. *NRC Handelsblad*, 14 April 2001.
209. *Nieuws* 2001, 3: 3.
210. Griffiths, Bood and Weyers 1998, footnotes 15 and 19.
211. Anaesthetist Admiraal and ethicist Dupuis respectively in the Dutch weekly *Elsevier* from 29 April 1989.
212. Jonquière 2002, 57: 505–7.
213. *Volkskrant*, 10 February 2001.
214. Handelingen Tweede Kamer, 2000–2001; 26691 and 22588, 42.
215. *NRC Handelsblad*, 10 April 2001.
216. Kelk 2001, speciaal nummer: 65–74, p. 73.
217. Both in the weekly *Elsevier*, 29 April 1989, p. 28.
218. *NRC Handelsblad*, 10 April 1993.
219. SCEN is an abbreviation for 'Steun en Consultatie Euthanasie Nederland' – Support and Consultation Euthanasia Netherlands.
220. Jonquière 2002, 57: 505–7.
221. Clark and Seymour 1999.
222. Rizzo 2000, 21: 277–89.
223. Clark 2002: 905–7.
224. Gordijn and Janssens 2000, 41: 35–6; Halper 2000: 81–116.
225. Jochemsen and Keown 1999, 25: 16–21.
226. Hoogerwerf 1999.
227. Drion 1992.
228. For an example of such an unfortunate turn of events, see Appendix I: Medical Disciplinary Court of Amsterdam, 14 January 1994.
229. Interview with the feministic monthly *Opzij*, February 1993.
230. *Nieuws* 2001, 3: 3.
231. Kennedy 2002.
232. Klotzko 1998: 398–406, p. 402.
233. Den Hartogh 2002, 26: 232–50.
234. Remmelink 2001, 19: 896.
235. Ten Have and Clark 2002.
236. Van Wijmen 1989.
237. Van der Maas, Delden and Pijnenborg 1991; Van der Wal and Van der Maas 1996; Van der Wal et al. 2003.

238. Admiraal 1992: 77–82.
239. Van der Wal et al. 2003, p. 99.
240. Ten Have and Janssens 2001; Janssens, Ten Have and Zylicz 1999, 25: 408–12.
241. Janssens 2001.
242. Block and Billings 2002, 154: 2039–47; Foley 1995, 4: 163–78.
243. Zylicz 1993, 4: 30–4.
244. Doyle, Hanks and MacDonald 1993, p. 3.
245. Van der Wal et al. 2003, p. 99.
246. Van der Wal and Van der Maas 1996, p. 56.
247. Government of the Netherlands 1997.
248. Francke, Persoon and Kerkstra 1997.
249. Bruntink 2002.
250. Zylicz 1994, 49: 139–40.

References

Achterhuis, H. (1980) *De markt van welzijn en geluk*. Baarn: Ambo.

Admiraal, P. V. (1992) A physician's responsibility to help a patient die, in R. I. Misbin (ed.) *Euthanasia: The Good of the Patient, The Good of Society*. Frederick, MD: University Publishing Group.

Aghina, M. J. (1978) *Patiëntenrecht. Een kwestie van gewicht*. Assen/Amsterdam: van Gorcum.

Arentz, D. H. (2001) Hulp bij zelfdoding, *Medisch Contact*, 56(9): 217–18.

Ariès, P. (1974) *Western Attitudes toward Death: From the Middle Ages to the Present*. Baltimore: Johns Hopkins University Press.

Ariès, P. (1981) *The Hour of Our Death*. New York: Knopf.

Ariès, P. (1985) *Images of Man and Death*. Cambridge: Cambridge University Press.

Becker, J. W. and Vink, R. (1994) *Secularisatie in Nederland, 1966–1991. De verandering van opvattingen en enkele gedragingen*. Rijswijk: Sociaal en Cultureel Planbureau.

Becker, J. W. and de Wit, J. S. J. (2000) *Secularisatie in de jaren negentig*. The Hague: Sociaal en Cultureel Planbureau.

Beemer, Th. (1977) Euthanasie: Moraaltheologische overwegingen, in P. Muntendam (ed.) *Euthanasie*. Leiden: Stafleu's Wetenschappelijke Uitgeverij.

Beemer, Th. (1986) Tegen een gehalveerde ethiek. In D. van Tol (ed.) *Euthanasie wetgeving: andere wegen*. Amsterdam: VU Uitgeverij.

Berg, J. H. van den (1956) *Metablectica of Leer der veranderingen. Beginselen van een historische psychologie*. Nijkerk: Callenbach.

Berg, J. H. van den (1959) *Het menselijk lichaam. I. Het geopende lichaam*. Nijkerk: Callenbach.

Berg, J. H. van den (1961) *Het menselijk lichaam II. Het verlaten lichaam*. Nijkerk: Callenbach.

Berg, J. H. van den (1969) *Medische Macht en Medische Ethiek*, 5 edn. Nijkerk: Callenbach.

Block, S. D. and Billings, J. A. (2002) Patient requests to hasten death: evaluation and management in terminal cases, *Archives of Internal Medicine*, 154: 2039–47.

Borst-Eilers, E. (1992) Euthanasia in the Netherlands: brief historical review and present situation, in R. I. Misbin (ed.) *Euthanasia: The Good of the Patient, The Good of Society*. Frederick, MD: University Publishing Group.

Bruntink, R. (2002) *Een goede plek om te sterven. Palliatieve zorg in Nederland. Een wegwijzer*. Zutphen/Apeldoorn: Plataan.

Buma, J. T. (1950) *De huisarts en zijn patient. Grondslagen van het medisch denken en handelen*. Amsterdam: Allert de Lange.

Buytendijk, F. J. J. (1947) *Het kennen van de innerlijkheid*. Nijmegen/Utrecht: Dekker & van de Vegt.

Buytendijk, F. J. J. (1959) De relatie arts-patiënt, *Nederlands Tijdschrift voor Geneeskunde*, 103: 2504–8.

CAL – Commissie Aanvaardbaarheid Levensbeëindigend Handelen KNMG (1997) *Medisch handelen rond het levenseinde bij wilsonbekwame patiënten*. Houten/Diegem: Bohn Stafleu van Loghum.

Chabot, B. E. (2001) *Sterfwerk. De dramaturgie van zelfdoding in eigen kring*. Nijmegen: SUN.

Clark, D. (2002) Between hope and acceptance: the medicalisation of dying, *British Medical Journal*, 324: 905–7.

Clark, D. and Seymour, J. (1999) *Reflections on Palliative Care*. Buckingham: Open University Press.

Dekker, G., de Hart, J. and Peters, J. (1997) *God in Nederland, 1966–1996*. Amsterdam: Anthos.

Dekkers, W. J. M. (2001) Images of death and dying, in H. A. M. J. ten Have and B. Gordijn (eds) *Bioethics in a European Perspective*. Dordrecht: Kluwer.

Delden, J. J. M. van (1993) *Beslissen om niet te reanimeren. Een medisch en ethisch vraagstuk*. Assen: van Gorcum.

Delden, J. J. M. van, Pijnenborg, L. and van der Maas, P. J. (1993) Dances with data, *Bioethics* 7(4): 323–9.

Dierick, G. (1983) *Vragen om de Dood: Beschouwingen over euthanasie*. Baarn: Ambo.

Dowbiggin, I. (2003) *A Merciful End. The Euthanasia Movement in Modern America*. New York: Oxford University Press.

Doyle, D., Hanks, G. W. C. and MacDonald, N. (1993) *Oxford Textbook on Palliative Medicine*. Oxford: Oxford University Press.

Drion, H. (1992) *Het zelfgewilde einde van oude mensen*. Amsterdam: Balans.

Dunning, A. J. (1981) *Broeder Ezel. Over het onvermogen in de geneeskunde*. Amsterdam/Utrecht: Meulenhoff/Wetenschappelijke Uitgeverij Bunge.

Dutch Catholic Bishops' Conference (2002) *Euthanasia and Human Dignity. A Collection of Contributions by the Dutch Catholic Bishops' Conference to the Legislative Procedure, 1983–2001*. Louvain: Uitgeverij Peeters.

Elias, N. (1985) *The Loneliness of the Dying*. Oxford: Blackwell.

Enthoven, L. (1987) *Op sterven na dood. Euthanasie in Nederland*. Utrecht/Antwerpen: Bohn, Scheltema & Holkema.

Enthoven, L. (1998) *Het recht op leven en dood*. Deventer: Kluwer.

Es, J. C. van (1974) Ieder sterft zijn eigen dood, in F. J. A. Huygen, P. Speth, C. P. Sporken and S. Swaans (eds) *Menswaardig sterven*. Bilthoven: Amboboeken.

Felling, A., Peters, J. and Schreuder, O. (1991) *Dutch Religion. The Religious Consciousness of The Netherlands after the Cultural Revolution.* Nijmegen: Instituut voor Toegepaste Sociale Wetenschappen.

Fenigsen, R. (1989) A case against Dutch euthanasia, *Hastings Center Report*, 19(1): S22–S30.

Foley, K. M. (1995) Pain, physician-assisted suicide and euthanasia, *Pain Forum* 4: 163–78.

Foucault, M. (1966) *Les mots et les choses.* Paris: Gallimard.

Francke, A. L., Persoon, A. and Kerkstra, A. (1997) *Palliatieve zorg in Nederland. Een inventarisatiestudie naar palliatieve zorg, deskundigheidsbevordering en zorg voor zorgenden.* Utrecht: NIVEL.

Galbraith, S. (1978) The 'no lose' philosophy in medicine, *Journal of Medical Ethics*, 4: 61–3.

Gezondheidsraad (1973) *Interim-advies inzake euthanasie.* The Hague: Gezondheidsraad.

Gezondheidsraad (1982a) *Advies inzake Euthanasie.* The Hague: Gezondheidsraad.

Gezondheidsraad (1982b) *Advies inzake Euthanasie bij Pasgeborenen.* The Hague: Gezondheidsraad.

Gezondheidsraad (1982c) *Advies inzake Euthanasie bij Pasgeborenen – Tweede interimadvies.* The Hague: Gezondheidsraad.

Gomez, C. F. (1991) Euthanasia: consider the Dutch, *Commonweal* 118(14, suppl.): 469–72.

Gordijn, B. (1998) Euthanasie: strafbar und doch zugestanden? Die niederländische Duldungspolitik in Sachen Euthanasie, *Ethik in der Medizin*, 10(1): 12–25.

Gordijn, B. and Janssens, R. (2000) The prevention of euthanasia through palliative care: new developments in The Netherlands, *Patient Education and Counseling*, 41: 35–6.

Government of the Netherlands (1997) *Standpunt van het kabinet naar aanleiding van de evaluatie van de meldingsprocedure euthanasie.* The Hague: SDU.

Griffiths, J., Bood, A. and Weyers, H. (1998) *Euthanasia and Law in The Netherlands.* Amsterdam: Amsterdam University Press.

Groenewoud, J. H., van der Heide, A., Onwuteaka-Philipsen, B., Willems, D. L., van der Maas, P. J. and van der Wal, G. (2000) Clinical problems with the performance of euthanasia and physician-assisted suicide in The Netherlands, *New England Journal of Medicine*, 342(8): 551–6.

Halman, L., Heunks, F., de Moor, R. and Zanders, H. (1987) *Traditie, secularisatie en individualisering. Een studie naar de waarden van de Nederlanders in een Europese context.* Tilburg: Tilburg University Press.

Halper, T. (2000) Accommodating death: euthanasia in The Netherlands, in H. T. Engelhardt (ed.) *The philosophy of medicine. Framing the field.* Dordrecht: Kluwer.

Hartogh, G. A. den (2002) Regulering van euthanasie en hulp bij suicide: hoe succesvol is het Nederlandse model?, *Tijdschrift voor Gezondheidsrecht*, 26(4): 232–50.

Have, H. A. M. J. ten (1995) The anthropological tradition in the philosophy of medicine, *Theoretical Medicine*, 16: 3–14.

Have, H. A. M. J. ten and Clark, D. (2002) *The Ethics of Palliative Care. European Perspectives.* Buckingham/Philadelphia: Open University Press.

Have, H. A. M. J. ten and Janssens, M. J. P. A. (1997) Regulating euthanasia in The Netherlands. Ethics committees for review of euthanasia?, *HEC (Healthcare Ethics Committee) Forum*, 94(4): 393–9.

Have, H. A. M. J. ten and Janssens, M. J. P. A. (2001) *Palliative Care in Europe. Concepts and Policies*. Amsterdam: IOS Press.

Have, H. A. M. J. ten and Welie, J. V. M. (1992) Euthanasia: normal medical practice?, *Hastings Center Report*, 22: 34–8.

Haverkate, I., Onwuteaka-Philipsen, B. D., van der Heide, A., Kostense, P. J., van der Wal, G. and van der Maas, P. J. (2001) Weigering van verzoeken om euthanasie of hulp bij zelfdoding meestal gebaseerd op ingeschatte niet-draaglijkheid van het lijden, de beschikbaarheid van behandelalternatieven en de aanwezigheid van depressieve klachten, *Nederlands Tijdschrift voor Geneeskunde*, 145(2): 80–4.

Hilhorst, H. (1983) *Euthanasie in het ziekenhuis*. Lochem/Poperinge: De Tijdstroom.

Hoofdakker, R. H. van den (1970) *Het bolwerk der beterweters*. Amsterdam: van Gennep.

Hoogerkamp, G. (1992) Euthanasie op het binnenhof. De euthanasiediscussie in politiek-historsich perspectief (1978–1992), *Utrechtse Historische Cahiers* 13(1).

Hoogerwerf, A. (1999) *Denken over sterven en dood in de geneeskunde*. Utrecht: van der Wees.

Huygen, F. J. A. (1978) *Family Medicine. The Medical Life History of Families*. Nijmegen: Dekker & van de Vegt.

Huysmans, F., Juffermans, P., Lagro, B., van Niekerk, B., Smits, F. and Vlaar, H. (1973) *Gezondheidszorg in Nederland*. Nijmegen: Socialistische Uitgeverij Nijmegen.

Illich, I. (1975) *Medical Nemesis: The Expropriation of Health*. London: Marion Boyars.

Indewey Gerlings-Huurman, T. (1977) *Het Leeuwarder euthanasie-proces. Feiten en commentaren*. Nijkerk: Callenbach.

Jacobs, F. C. L. M. (1990) Medisch zinloos handelen en zinloos medisch handelen, *Medisch Contact*, 45(17): 541–3.

Jannink-Kappelle, W. W. (1992) Euthanasieverklaring/weigering behandeling; nieuwe tekst Nederlandse Vereniging voor Vrijwillige Euthanasie, *Medisch Contact*, 47: 845–7.

Janssens, M. J. P. A. (2001) *Palliative Care: Concepts and Ethics*. Nijmegen: Nijmegen University Press.

Janssens, M. J. P. A., ten Have, H. A. M. J. and Zylicz, Z. (1999) Hospice and euthanasia in The Netherlands: an ethical point of view, *Journal of Medical Ethics*, 25: 408–12.

Jochemsen, H. and Keown, J. (1999) Voluntary euthanasia under control? Further empirical evidence from The Netherlands, *Journal of Medical Ethics*, 25: 16–21.

Jonquière, R. (2002) Euthanasie als exportproduct, *Medisch Contact*, 57(13): 505–7.

Juffermans, P. (1982) *Staat en gezondheidszorg in Nederland*. Nijmegen: Socialistische Uitgeverij Nijmegen.

Kelk, C. (2001) Nieuwe contouren van toelaatbare euthanasie, *Tijdschrift voor Gezondheidsrecht*, speciaal nummer: 65–74.

Kennedy, J. (2002) *Een weloverwogen dood. Euthanasie in Nederland*. Amsterdam: Uitgeverij Bert Bakker.

Kenter, E. G. H. (1983) Euthanasie in een huisartsenpraktijk, *Medisch Contact*, 38: 1179–82.

Keown, J. (1995) Euthanasia in The Netherlands: sliding down the slippery slope?, in J. Keown (ed.) *Euthanasia Examined: Ethical, Clinical and Legal Perspectives*. New York: Cambridge University Press.

Klijn, A., Otlowski, M. and Trappenburg, M. (2001) *Regulating Physician-Negotiated Death*. The Hague: Elsevier.

Klijn, W. C. M. and Nieboer, W. (1984) *Euthanasie en hulp bij zelfdoding – ethische analyse en waardering – wet en recht*. Utrecht: Katholieke Vereniging van Ziekeninrichtingen.

Klotzko, A. J. (1997) An embryonic dilemma, *Nursing Times*, 93: 38–9.

Klotzko, A. J. (1998) What kind of life? What kind of death? An Interview with Dr Henk Prins, in D. C. Thomasma, T. Kimbrough-Kushner, G. K. Kimsma and C. Ciesielkski-Carlucci (eds) *Asking to Die. Inside the Dutch Debate about Euthanasia*. Dordrecht: Kluwer.

Klotzko, A. J. and Chabot, B. E. (1998) Assisted suicide in the absence of somatic illness, in D. C. Thomasma, T. Kimbrough-Kushner, G. K. Kimsma and C. Ciesielkski-Carlucci (eds) *Asking to Die. Inside the Dutch Debate about Euthanasia*. Dordrecht: Kluwer.

KNMG – Koninklijke Nederlandsche Maatschappij tot Bevordering der Geneeskunst (1936) *Medische ethiek*. Amsterdam: KNMG.

KNMG – Koninklijke Nederlandsche Maatschappij tot Bevordering der Geneeskunst (1959) *Medische ethiek en gedragsleer*. Amsterdam: KNMG.

KNMG – Koninklijke Nederlandse Maatschappij tot Bevordering der Geneeskunst (1984) Standpunt inzake euthanasie, *Medisch Contact*, 31: 990–1002.

KNMG – Koninklijke Nederlandse Maatschappij tot Bevordering der Geneeskunst (1997) Reactie van het Hoofdbestuur op het kabinetsstandpunt uit januari 1997, *Medisch Contact*, 53(13): 420–25.

Kolfschoten, F. van (2003) Dutch television report stirs up euthanasia controversy, *Lancet*, 361: 1352–3.

Kooyman, F. C. (1959) 'Reanimatie', aanwinst, probleem en opgave, *Medisch Contact*, 14: 441–4.

Kübler-Ross, L. (1969) *On Death and Dying*. New York: Macmillan.

Kuhn, T. S. (1962) *The Structure of Scientific Revolutions*. Chicago: University of Chicago Press.

Kuitert, H. M. (1981) *Een gewenste dood – euthanasie en zelfbeschikking als moreel en godsdienstig probleem*. Baarn: Ten Have.

Kuitert, H. M. (1993) *Mag er een einde komen aan het bittere einde?* Baarn: Ten Have.

Leenen, H. J. J. (1977) Euthanasie in het gezondheidsrecht, in P. Muntendam (ed.) *Euthanasie*. Leiden: Stafleu.

Leenen, H. J. J. (1978) Recht op eigen lichaam, *Tijdschrift voor Gezondheidsrecht*, 2: 1–8.

Legemate, J. (1998) 25 jaar euthanasie-beleid: tijd voor legalisering, *Tijdschrift voor*

Geneeskunde en Ethiek, 8: 14–20.

Lindeboom, G. A. (1979) The physicians' oath of the Friesian University in Franeker (1640), *Nederlands Tijdschrift voor Geneeskunde*, 123: 1610–11.

Maas, P. J. van der, van Delden, J. J. M. and Pijnenborg, L. (1991) *Medische Beslissingen Rond het Levenseinde.* Amsterdam: Sdu Uitgeverij.

McWhinney, I. R. (1989) *A Textbook of Family Medicine.* New York/Oxford: Oxford University Press.

Matse, J. (1974) De nieuwe dood, in F. J. A. Huygen, P. Speth, C. P. Sporken and S. Swaans (eds) *Menswaardig sterven.* Bilthoven: Amboboeken.

Meerman, D. (1991) *Goed doen door dood te maken. Een analyse van de morele argumentatie in vijf maatschappelijke debatten over euthanasie tussen 1870 en 1940 in Engeland en Duitsland.* Kampen: Kok.

Menges, J. (1972) *'Euthanasie' in het Derde Rijk.* Haarlem: De Erven F. Bohn.

Mertens, A. (1960) Concrete handelwijze in de Nederlandse katholieke ziekenhuizen, *R. K. Artsenblad*, 39: 94–100.

Meulenbelt, J. (1986) Brief aan de regering n. a. v. het rapport van de Staatscommissie Euthanasia, *Vita Humana: Tijdschrift voor Medische Ethiek*, 13(1): 7–14.

Meyler, L. (1973) Euthanasie, *Nederlands Tijdschrift voor Geneeskunde*, 117: 553–5.

Muntendam, P. (1977) Verantwoording en inleiding euthanasie, in P. Muntendam (ed.) *Euthanasie.* Leiden: Stafleu.

NVK – Nederlandse Vereniging voor Kindergeneeskunde (1992) *Doen of laten: Grenzen van het medisch handelen in de neonatologie.* Utrecht: NVK.

NVP – Nederlandse Vereniging voor Psychiatrie (1992) Mededelingen bestuur, *Nieuws en Mededelingen*, 86(2): 2–3.

NVVE – Nederlandse Vereniging voor Vrijwillige Euthanasie (1991) *Voorstel voor een Euthanasieprotocol.* Amsterdam: NVVE.

NVVE – Nederlandse Vereniging voor Vrijwillige Euthanasie (1992) Euthanasieverklaring/weigering behandeling, *Medisch Contact*, 47(27–8): 846–7.

Onwuteaka-Philipsen, B. (1999) *Consultation of Another Physician in Cases of Euthanasia and Physician-assisted Suicide.* Amsterdam: Free University of Amsterdam.

Orie, N. G. (1968) Aanvaarding of Verwerping, *Nederlands Tijdschrift voor Geneeskunde*, 112: 1832–6.

Otter, G. den (1968) De betekenis van de huidige geneeskunde voor de mens van vandaag, *Medisch Contact*, 23: 846–50.

Peursen, C. A. van (1968) Gevolgen voor patiënt, arts en gemeenschap van de recente vorderingen in de geneeskunde, *Nederlands Tijdschrift voor Geneeskunde*, 112: 1814–18.

Ponsioen, B. P. (1983) Hoe leert de huisarts leven met euthanasie?, *Nederlands Tijdschrift voor Geneeskunde*, 127: 961–4.

Pool, R. (2000) *Negotiating a Good Death. Euthanasia in The Netherlands.* New York/London/Oxford: Haworth Press.

Proctor, R. N. (1988) *Racial Hygiene: Medicine under the Nazis.* Cambridge, MA: Harvard University Press.

Ree, F. van der (2001) Genoeg van het leven, *Medisch Contact*, 56(11): 426–8.

Regionale Toetsingscommissies Euthanasie (2000) *Jaarverslag 1998/1999.* The

Hague: Ministry of Justice.
Regionale Toetsingscommissies Euthanasie (2001) *Jaarverslag 2000*. The Hague: Ministry of Justice.
Regionale Toetsingscommissies Euthanasie (2002) *Jaarverslag 2001*. The Hague: Ministry of Justice.
Regionale Toetsingscommissies Euthanasie (2003) *Jaarverslag 2002*. The Hague: Ministry of Justice.
Remmelink, J. (1996) *Mr. D. Hazewinkel-Suringa's Inleiding tot de studie van het Nederlands strafrecht*, 15 edn. Deventer: Gouda Quint.
Remmelink, J. (2001) Moord en euthanasie, *Nederlands Juristenblad*, 19: 896.
Rigter, R. B. M. (1992) *Met raad en daad. De geschiedenis van de Gezondheidsraad 1902–1985*. Rotterdam: Erasmus Publishing.
Rizzo, R. F. (2000) Physician-assisted suicide in the United States: the underlying factors in technology, health care and palliative medicine, *Theoretical Medicine and Bioethics*, 21: 277–89.
Salomon, A. (1948) *Arts en patient. Een ethische en psychologische leidraad*. Amsterdam: Wetenschappelijke Uitgeverij.
SCP – Sociaal en Cultureel Planbureau (2002) *Sociale en Culturele Verkenningen*. Rijswijk: SCP.
Spaink, K. (2001) *De dood in doordrukstrip*. Amsterdam: Nijgh & van Ditmaar.
Sporken, P. (1969) *Voorlopige diagnose. Inleiding tot een medische ethiek*. Bilthoven: Amboboeken.
Sporken, P. (1977) *Ethiek en Gezondheidszorg*. Baarn: Amboboeken.
Sporken, P. (1981) *Heb jij aanvaard dat ik sterven moet? – stervenden en hun helpers*. Baarn: Ambo.
Staatscommissie Euthanasie (1985) *Rapport van de Staatscommissie Euthanasie – Advies – Deel 1*. The Hague: SDU.
Terborgh-Dupuis, H. (1976) *Medische ethiek in perspectief. Een onderzoek naar normen en argumentaties in de (medische) ethiek*. Leiden: Stafleu's Wetenschappelijke Uitgeversmaatschappij.
The, A. M. (1997) *'vanavond om 8 uur ...' Verpleegkundige dilemma's bij euthanasie en andere beslissingen rond het levenseinde*. Houtem/Diegem: Bohn Stafleu van Loghum.
Thomasma, D. C., Kimbrough-Kushner, T., Kimsma, G. K. and Ciesielski-Carlucci, C. (1998) *Asking to Die. Inside the Dutch Debate about Euthanasia*. Dordrecht: Kluwer.
Thung, P. J. (1966) *Wat is er gaande in de geneeskunde?* Leiden: Universitaire Pers.
Veatch, R. M. (1978) Codes of medical ethics: ethical analysis, in W. T. Reich (ed.) *Encyclopedia of Bioethics*. New York: Free Press.
Veldhuis, R. (1988) Tired of living, afraid of dying: reflections on the practice of euthanasia in The Netherlands, *Studies in Christian Ethics*, 11(1): 63–7.
Wachter, R. M. (1992) AIDS, activism, and the politics of health, *New England Journal of Medicine*, 326(2): 128–33.
Wal, G. van der (1992) *Euthanasie en hulp bij zelfdoding door huisartsen*. Rotterdam: WYT Uitgeefgroep.
Wal, G. van der and van der Maas, P. J. (1996) *Euthanasie en andere beslissingen rond het levenseinde. De praktijk en de meldingsprocedure*. The Hague: SDU.
Wal, G. van der, van Eijk, J. Th. M., Leenen, H. J. J. and Spreeuwenberg, C. (1991a)

Euthanasie en hulp bij zelfdoding door huisartsen. Een onderzoek: opzet en methode, *Medisch Contact*, 46(6): 171–3.

Wal, G. van der, van Eijk, J. Th. M., Leenen, H. J. J. and Spreeuwenberg, C. (1991b) Euthanasie en hulp bij zelfdoding door huisartsen. Hoe gaan huisartsen om met de inhoudelijke zorgvuldigheidseisen, *Medisch Contact*, 46(7): 211–15.

Wal, G. van der, van Eijk, J. Th. M., Leenen, H. J. J. and Spreeuwenberg, C. (1991c) Euthanasie en hulp bij zelfdoding door huisartsen. Hoe vaak komt dit feitelijk voor, *Medisch Contact*, 46(6): 174–6.

Wal, G. van der, van Eijk, J. Th. M., Leenen, H. J. J. and Spreeuwenberg, C. (1991d) Euthanasie en hulp bij zelfdoding door huisartsen. Procedurele zorgvuldigheidseisen, *Medisch Contact*, 46(8): 237–45.

Wal, G. van der, van der Maas, P. J. and Bosma, J. M. (1996) Evaluation of the notification procedure for physician-assisted death in The Netherlands, *New England Journal of Medicine*, 335: 1706–11.

Wal, G. A. van der, van der Heide, A., Onwuteaka-Philipsen, B. and van der Maas, P. J. (2003) *Medische besluitvorming aan het einde van het leven. De praktijk en de toetsingsprocedure euthanasie.* Utrecht: De Tijdstroom.

Weizsäcker, V. von (1950) Grundfragen medizinischer Anthropologie, in V. von Weizsäcker (ed.) *Diesseits und Jenseits der Medizin.* Stuttgart: K. F. Köhler.

Welie, J. V. M. (1992) The medical exception: physicians, euthanasia and the Dutch criminal law, *Journal of Medicine and Philosophy*, 17(4): 419–37.

Welie, J. V. M. (2001) Living wills and substituted judgments: a critical analysis, *Medicine, Health Care and Philosophy*, 4(2): 169–83.

Welie, J. V. M. (2002) Why physicians? Reflections on The Netherlands' new euthanasia law, *Hastings Center Report*, 32(1): 42–4.

Welie, J. V. M. (2004) The tendency of contemporary decision making strategies to deny the condition of Alzheimer disease, in R. B. Purtilo and H. A. M. J. ten Have (eds) *Ethical Foundations of Palliative Care for Alzheimer Disease.* Baltimore: John Hopkins University Press, 163–180.

Weyers, H. (2002) *Euthanasie: het proces van rechtsverandering.* Groningen: University of Groningen.

Wibaut, F. P. (2001) De willekeur van het Openbaar Ministerie. Stervenshulp als onderwerp van juridische scherpslijperij, *Medisch Contact*, 56(17): 657–9.

Wijmen, F. C. B. van (1989) *Artsen en het zelfgekozen levenseinde. Verslag van een onderzoek onder artsen naar opvattingen en gedragingen ten aanzien van euthanasie en hulp bij zelfdoding.* Maastricht: University of Maastricht (Limburg), Department of Health Law.

Wortman, J. L. C. (1929) *De ethica aan het ziekbed.* Haarlem: De Erven F. Bohn.

Zola, I. K. (1972) The medicalizing of society, *Huisarts en Wetenschap*, 15: 229–30.

Zola, I. K. (1973) *De medische macht.* Meppel: Boom.

Zylicz, Z. (1993) Hospice in Holland. The story behind the blank spot, *American Journal of Hospice and Palliative Care*, 4: 30–4.

Zylicz, Z. (1994) Ondersteuning van de thuiszorg voor terminale patiënten: Hospice Rozenheuvel, *Medisch Contact*, 49: 139–40.

Zylicz, Z. and Janssens, M. J. P. A. (1998) Options in palliative care: dealing with those who want to die, *Baillière's Clinical Anaesthesiology*, 12(1): 121–31.

Index

THE ETHICS OF PALLIATIVE CARE

European Perspectives

Henk ten Have and David Clark (eds)

As palliative care develops across many of the countries of Europe, we find that it continues to raise important ethical challenges. Palliative care practice requires ethical sensitivity and understanding. At the same time the very existence of palliative care calls for ethical explanation. Ethics and palliative care meet over some vital issues: 'the good death', sedation at the end of life, requests for euthanasia, futile treatment, and the role of research. Yet palliative care appears uncertain about its goals and there is evidence that its ethical underpinnings are changing. Likewise, the moral problems of palliative care are only partly served by the four 'principles' of modern bioethics. This innovative book, with contributions by clinicians, ethicists, philosophers and social scientists, provides the first ever picture of palliative care ethics in the European context. It will be of interest to those involved in the delivery and management of palliative care services, as well as to students and researchers.

Contents: *Series editor's preface – Introduction: the work of the Pallium Project –* **Part one: Concepts and Models of Care** *– Introduction to Part one – Palliative care and the historical background – Palliative care developments in seven European countries – Conceptual tensions in European palliative care –* **Part two: Moral Values** *– Introduction to Part two – Moral values in palliative care: a European comparison – From conviction to responsibility in palliative care ethics – Good death or good life as a goal of palliative care – Palliative care: a relational approach –* **Part three: Ethics and Palliative Care Practice** *– Introduction to Part three – Respect for autonomy and palliative care – Sedation in palliative care: facts and concepts – Euthanasia and physician assisted suicide – Research ethics and palliative care – Futility, limits and palliative care – Conclusion – References – Index.*

272pp   0 335 21140 2 (Paperback)   0 335 21141 0 (Hardback)

A GOOD DEATH
On the Value of Death and Dying

Lars Sandman

- Is there such a thing as a good death?
- Should we be able to choose how we wish to die?
- What are the ethical considerations that surround a good death?

The notion of a 'good death' plays an important role in modern palliative care but remains a topic for lively debate. Using philosophical methods and theories, this book provides a critical analysis of Western notions surrounding the dying process in the palliative care context. Sandman highlights how our changing ideas about the value of life inevitably shape the concept of a good death. He explores the varying perspectives on the good death that come from friends, family, physicians, spiritual carers and others close to the dying person. Setting out a number of arguments for and against existing thinking about a good death, this book links to the practice of palliative care in several key areas:

- An exploration of the universal features of dying
- The process of facing death
- Preparation for death
- The environment of dying and death

The author concludes that it is difficult to find convincing reasons for any one way to die a good death and argues for a pluralist approach.

A Good Death is essential reading for students and professionals with an interest in palliative care and end-of-life issues.

Contents: *Series editor's preface – Acknowledgements – Introduction – Ethics and value – Death, dying and beyond – Global features of death and dying – Facing death – Prepared to die – The environment of dying and death – Ideas about good dying within palliative care – Bibliography – Index.*

184pp   0 335 21411 8 (Paperback)   0 335 21412 6 (Hardback)

LOSS, CHANGE AND BEREAVEMENT IN PALLIATIVE CARE
Pam Firth, Gill Luff and David Oliviere

- How do professionals meet the needs of bereaved people?
- How do professionals undertake best practice with individuals, groups, families and communities?
- What are the implications for employing research to influence practice?

This book provides a resource for working with a complex range of loss situations and includes chapters on childhood bereavement, and individual and family responses to loss and change. It contains the most up-to-date work in the field presented by experienced practitioners and researchers and is relevant not only for those working in specialist palliative care settings, but for professionals in general health and social care sectors.

Strong links are maintained between research and good practice throughout the book. These are reinforced by the coherent integration of international research material and the latest thinking about loss and bereavement. Experts and clinicians draw upon their knowledge and practice, whilst the essential perspective of the service user is central to this book.

Loss, Change and Bereavement in Palliative Care provides essential reading for a range of professional health and social care disciplines practising at postgraduate or post-registration/qualification level. It challenges readers, at an advanced level, on issues of loss, change and bereavement.

Contributors:
Lesley Adshead, Jenny Altschuler, Peter Beresford, Grace H. Christ, Suzy Croft, Pam Firth, Shirley Firth, Richard Harding, Felicity Hearn, Jennie Lester, Gill Luff, Linda Machin, Jan McLaren, David Oliviere, Ann Quinn, Phyllis R. Silverman, Jean Walker, Karen Wilman.

Contents: *Notes on the contributors – Series editor's preface – Acknowledgements – Foreword – Introduction – The context of loss, change and bereavement in palliative care – Mourning: a changing view – Research in practice – Illness and loss within the family – Life review with the terminally ill – narrative therapies – The death of a child – Interventions with bereaved children – Involving service users in palliative care: from theory to practice – Excluded and vulnerable groups of service users – Carers: current research and developments – Groupwork in palliative care – Cultural perspectives on loss and bereavement – Conclusions – Index.*

240pp   0 335 21323 5 (Paperback)   0 335 21324 3 (Hardback)

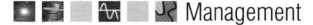
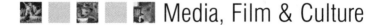
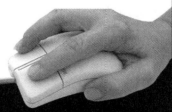